Introduction to Evidence-Based Practice in Nursing and Health Care

Edited by
Kathy Malloch, PhD, MBA, RN, FAAN
President of Malloch & Associates
Arizona State University

Tim Porter-O'Grady, PhD, EdD, RN, FAAN
Senior Partner of Tim Porter-O'Grady Associates
Emory University

JONES AND BARTLETT PUBLISHERS
Sudbury, Massachusetts
BOSTON   TORONTO   LONDON   SINGAPORE

World Headquarters

Jones and Bartlett Publishers
40 Tall Pine Drive
Sudbury, MA 01776
978-443-5000
info@jbpub.com
www.jbpub.com

Jones and Bartlett Publishers
Canada
6339 Ormindale Way
Mississauga, ON L5V 1J2
CANADA

Jones and Bartlett Publishers
International
Barb House, Barb Mews
London W6 7PA
UK

Jones and Bartlett's books and products are available through most bookstores and online book-sellers. To contact Jones and Bartlett Publishers directly, call 800-832-0034, fax 978-443-8000, or visit our website www.jbpub.com.

Substantial discounts on bulk quantities of Jones and Bartlett's publications are available to cor-porations, professional associations, and other qualified organizations. For details and specific dis-count information, contact the special sales department at Jones and Bartlett via the above contact information or send an email to specialsales@jbpub.com.

ISBN-13: 978-0-7637-2913-4
ISBN-10: 0-7637-2913-2

Library of Congress Cataloging-in-Publication Data

Introduction to evidence-based practice in nursing and health care / [edited by] Kathy Malloch, Tim Porter-O'Grady.
  p. ; cm.
  Includes bibliographical references.
  ISBN 0-7637-2913-2
  1. Evidence-based nursing. 2. Evidence-based medicine.
  [DNLM: 1. Evidence-Based Medicine. 2. Nursing Care. 3. Nursing Research.] I. Malloch, Kathy.
II. Porter-O'Grady, Timothy.
  RT42.I584 2006
  610.73—dc22
6048   2005004503

Production Credits

Acquisitions Editor: Kevin Sullivan
Associate Editor: Amy Sibley
Production Director: Amy Rose
Production Editor: Renée Sekerak
Production Assistant: Rachel Rossi
Marketing Manager: Emily Ekle
Manufacturing Buyer: Therese Connell
Composition: Auburn Associates, Inc.
Cover Design: Kristin E. Ohlin
Printing and Binding: Malloy Incorporated
Cover Printing: Malloy Incorporated

Printed in the United States of America
10 09 08 07 06   10 9 8 7 6 5 4 3 2

Contents

Chapter 6. The Journey to Evidence: Managing the Information
Infrastructure 125
Robert C. Geibert

Chapter 7. Managing Variance Through an Evidence-Based Framework
for Safe and Reliable Health Care 149
Kathy A. Scott

Contributors

Virginia Trotter Betts, RN, MSN, JD, FAAN
Commissioner for Policy
Tennessee Department of Mental Health and Developmental Disability

Karen Butler, MSN, RN
Lecturer and Clinical Instructor
College of Nursing
University of Kentucky

Rosalyn Cama, FASID
President
CAMA, Inc.
Chair of the Board, Center for Health Design

Susan R. Cooper, MSN, RN
Assistant Dean of Faculty Practice
Assistant Professor
Vanderbilt University School of Nursing

Marie P. Farrell, MPH, RN, FAAN
Professor and Chairperson
Department of Nursing
California State University, Bakersfield

Marcia K. Flesner, PhD, RN
Clinical Educator
Sinclair School of Nursing
University of Missouri-Columbia

Robert C. Geibert, EdD, RN
Senior Management Consultant
ACS Healthcare Services

Jill Gentry
Special Assistant to the Commissioner
Tennessee Department of Mental Health and Developmental Disability

Diane Heliker, PhD, RN
Associate Professor
Interim Associate Dean for Research
School of Nursing
University of Texas Medical Branch

Kathy Malloch, PhD, MBA, RN, FAAN
President
Kathy Malloch & Associates
Arizona State University

Roxanne McDaniel, PhD, RN
Associate Dean
Sinclair School of Nursing
University of Missouri-Columbia

Louise Miller, PhD, RN
Assistant Professor of Clinical Nursing
Sinclair School of Nursing
University of Missouri-Columbia

Tim Porter-O'Grady, PhD, EdD, RN,
    FAAN
Senior Partner
Tim Porter-O'Grady Associates
Emory University

Marilyn Rantz, PhD, RN, FAAN
Professor
Sinclair School of Nursing
University of Missouri-Columbia

Dolora C. Sanares, RN, MPA
Program Manager for Evidence-Based
    Practice
Nursing Practice and Professional
    Advancement
University of Texas Medical Branch

Elaine Scherer, RN, MA, BSN, RN
Director
American Nurses Credentialing Center
Magnet Recognition Program

Kathy A. Scott, PhD, RN
Chief Nursing Officer/Associate Ad-
    ministrator
Banner Thunderbird Medical Center

Amy Steinbinder, PhD, RN, CNA
Administrator
Safety and Innovation
Magnet Program Appraiser
Banner Thunderbird Medical Center

Preface

In an ideal world, the expenditure of energy, time, and money results in corresponding value that is clearly evident to both the giver and the receiver of the energy, time, and money. Evidence of the relationship between the expenditure of resources and the value to the recipient is readily apparent and appreciated. However, this new world of information has seriously challenged the allocation of resources and the basis from which future decisions are made. Consumers are not content to expend resources for undefined and unpredictable results. Clear evidence linking expenditures to outcomes that provide value given limited human, physical, and financial resources is essential for survival and sustainability.

Interestingly, expectations for outcome value linked to resource expenditures has not been a priority or an expectation in health care. The marketplace has focused on access to health care and financial coverage for citizens without a linkage to value-based outcomes. Health care workers, particularly nurses, have yet to fully identify and articulate the value consumers receive for the time and energy that nurses expend, the fiscal support provided by the marketplace for those services, and the specific relationships between those resources expended and value received.

Nurses, as both providers of health care services and consumers, are well positioned to not only improve the economic status of health care expenditures, but also to advance the science of evidence-based resource allocation through the advancement of evidence-based practice in nursing. The continuing evolution of world complexity in the age of technology presents new challenges and expectations for the profession of nursing. In fact, producing evidence of value in practice cannot be achieved without engaging a level of digital technology that simply has not as yet been fully engaged and invested in by the health care system. Increasing consumer involvement in health care services and the expectation of evidence that value does indeed result from the fiscal resources expended is the reality. Never before have the challenges been so motivating for nursing and the potential so significant for the explication of its value. During the last ten years, nursing has embraced and begun to integrate the gold standard of health care—evidence-based practice (EBP)—to advance the profession of nursing. Never in the history of nursing has there been a better time for the nursing professional to be recognized for the differences made in the health care system and in the outcomes of individual patient services. Creating evidence will serve to validate and document the value of nursing practice, and doing so is also a call to celebrate the incredible value and efficacy of nursing. This compelling opportunity is much more than a mere invitation. It is a mandate for the profession to continue the journey initiated by Florence Nightingale.

To be sure, the journey is not only transformational, it requires the involvement of all forces impacting the world of nursing practice. This book provides an overview of the world of evidence for nursing practice and includes application of the EBP principles presented from differing perspectives, thus combining theoretical underpinnings and real world experience from experts with practical application to the practice of nursing. Specifically, the governance structure, organizational vision and values, goals, allocation of resources, implications for technology, educational processes, support for staff nurse clinical excellence, management of errors using high reliability theory, workload management systems embedded in the reality of the marketplace, and evaluation for excellence using the Magnet framework are presented as a broad overview of the far reaching implications for evidence in an integrated, highly interconnected health care system. In addition, barriers to the integration of an evidentiary approach to nursing are discussed as well as strategies to overcome those barriers.

Closing the gap between evidence and practice requires knowledge, commitment, resilience, and a belief that this is the right course to explicate the essence of nursing and to further embed the value of nursing in the marketplace. As always, this work is a journey and not a destination. Your comments and suggestions to further enhance this work are encouraged and welcomed.

Kathy Malloch and Tim Porter-O'Grady

Acknowledgments

The collective wisdom of the contributing authors of this text offers not only the essence of evidence-based practice; the best research available, expertise of the practitioners, the values of those involved, but also many thought provoking and innovative challenges to enhance the journey of nursing practice that is based on evidence. We are deeply grateful for the collective expertise of this work that offers a single source of information for 10 critical areas of nursing practice that impact a large majority of the country's 2.8 million nurses.

Each chapter author provides significant insight and depth in the discussion as well as demonstrates their passion for each topic. Our colleagues have shared their wisdom, their passion, and their very precious time in the preparation of these chapters. We have both learned much from each of the chapters and continue to marvel at the incredible knowledge and willingness of each author to contribute their special expertise to the evidence-based practice knowledge reference for other nurses. To be sure, no one nurse can know it all and it is only through their generosity that the profession of nursing evolves and advances its science.

Thank you to our authors....

To Dolly Sanares and Dr. Diane Heliker for their willingness to share their model of Disciplined Clinical Inquiry (DCI), the ultimate application of evidence-based practice principles in the practice setting that was developed in collaboration with the University of Texas Medical Branch at Galveston.

To Dr. Bob Geibert for his creative and thorough review of the literature specific to technology and the electronic health record. His insight and ability to present the complex issues and challenges of the management of computerized information is a gift for those of us who struggle with integrating the work of nursing into the world of technology.

To Dr. Marie Farrell for her wisdom and rich overview of the challenges of information synthesis. Her global perspective offers a new lens for analysis and integration of the science of nursing into practice.

To Dr. Amy Steinbinder and Elaine Scherer for taking the risk to go above and beyond the norm in the development of the chapter on evidence for magnet accreditation. As their first official book chapter, the results reflect that of experienced and competent writers.

To Dr. Kathy Scott for her willingness to share her recent dissertation findings and evolving expertise in the area of patient safety and high reliability organizations. Her work is essential reading in this time of great emphasis on patient safety.

To Roz Cama, nationally recognized architect for creating healing spaces. She has brought this body of knowledge to a new level in documenting the link between physical space design, color, light, and nature and the processes of healing in addition to the creation of space that support the work of nursing in a safe and ergonomically sound manner.

To Drs. Marcia Flesner, Louise Miller, Roxanne McDaniel, and Marilyn Rantz, educators and innovators who continually push the walls of learning and practice advancement. Their insights into the need for and encouragement of evidence-based practices in learning and leading in clinical practice challenge us to think deeply and differently about the future of learning.

Ginna Betts and colleagues Susan Cooper, Karen Butler, and Jill Gentry who work tirelessly to meet the needs of the health of the community and challenge their nursing and health colleagues to demonstrate a commitment to advocacy, meeting the needs of the marginalized, and making sure that we are actually improving the health of those we serve.

Finally, our own work on governance, workload management, and building preferred health models for the future is designed to provide new and innovative strategies for understanding current challenges, evaluating available evidence, and continuing to develop new skills in asking better questions about our work that will open the doors to new models and structures for evidence-based practice.

Kathy Malloch and Tim Porter-O'Grady

CHAPTER 1

A New Age for Practice: Creating the Framework for Evidence

Tim Porter-O'Grady

Evidence-based practice is simply the integration of the best possible research to evidence with clinical expertise and with patient needs. Patient needs in this case refer specifically to the expectations, concerns, and requirements that patients bring to their clinical experience. It seems unusual that evidence-based practice should be discussed at all. Certainly, in the professional practice of health care, it should be easily concluded that practitioners want to provide only that care that makes a positive difference in the lives of those whom they serve. However, the history of medical practice and nursing care does not well represent either a methodology or process specifically devoted to achieving the best therapeutic procedures and clinical practice (Sackett, Straus, Richardson, Rosenberg, & Haynes, 2000).

It is only in the past decade that technology has made it possible for practitioners to begin to focus on collecting sufficient data to determine the best approach to clinical practice. Using digital means, huge components and aggregates of clinical information can now be integrated, compared, and contrasted in a way that reveals significant valuable information. It is this information and the knowledge it generates with regard to decision-making that provide a critical framework for systematic evidence-based clinical practice (Mazurek, Melnyk, & Fineout-Overholt, 2004).

The use of evidence-based practice requires an integration of individual clinical applications with the best available and current external clinical evidence. This evidence is drawn from a systematic exploration of the available relevant data and their applicability to an individual clinical circumstance (Figure 1.1). Individual clinical expertise requires a level of proficiency of judgment that has been acquired through both formal education and life experience. Learning occurs through formal and informal means, which provide a frame of reference that will ultimately inform and influence practice. "Experience simply means the amount of time and effort that is devoted to un-

Figure 1.1   The Keystones of Evidence

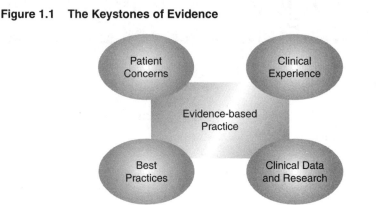

dertaking specified clinical activities in a way that results in expertise in their application" (Law, 2002, p. 3).

On the other hand, external clinical evidence reflects a body of clinically relevant data drawn from a variety of related sources that have a direct impact and meaning for specific clinical practice. External data are often based on precise clinical research that can be directly related to the specific clinical circumstances or processes under consideration. External clinical evidence can either validate or invalidate previous clinical experience and applications depending on the efficacy, power, accuracy, and applicability of the data with regard to specific clinical circumstances.

Sound practitioners depend both on solid clinical experience and good clinical data. In evidence-based processes, both extensive clinical experience and strong clinical research have validity, and when combined, they create and promote a strong argument for sustaining specific clinical practices. The unique element of evidence-based practice is that it is not specifically an academic or research exercise. Because of its connection to the practical application of care, evidence-based practice provides a strong validity and a firm foundation upon which to build clinical activities, and draw from them specific elements that contribute to explicitly defined health outcomes. Through modalities of evidence-based practice, the clinician can develop a realistic set of tools that, when applied and replicated, can produce continuing and valid clinical outcomes within the context of specific clinical circumstances (Muir, 2001).

Many practitioners are concerned about evidence-based practice, often describing it as "cookie cutter" or "cookbook" clinical practice. Nothing could be further from the truth. Evidence-based practice is generated from the practice setting, guided by practitioners, and represents the aggregation and integration of actual applied clinical experience in the generation of objective data through practice-based processes and methodologies (Breslin & Lucas, 2003). At the same time, evidence-based practice respects and, indeed, includes the vagaries of individual human circumstances and applications that frequently call for adjustment and change in practice. Introduction of human variability becomes one of the elements of evidence requiring accommodation as a part of the value of applying evidence-based practice within specific clinical settings. This match between external and objective clinical data and applied subjective clinical judgment is one of the critical clinical values for an evidence-based practice. Operating out of this framework ensures that specific clinical practice is not only relevant and based on the best available knowledge, but is also adaptive, reflecting the particular needs of individual patients as reflected in good clinical decision-making.

Clinical practitioners frequently suggest that evidence-based practice is used as a means for justifying cost cutting and resource reduction. Some believe that evidence-based practice would simply aid the nonclinical money managers in reducing resources so that clinical efficacy can be sacrificed on the altar of profitability. Furthermore, many clinical practitioners fear that these financial regulators will hold them hostage to specific clinical practices that tend to favor cost reduction rather than quality performance and, thus, cause them to fail to act in the best interests of the patient. Of course, this would be a profound misuse of the processes of evidence-based practice as well as wholly unethical and clinically inappropriate.

> **Evidence-based practice is not a cookbook or cookie-cutter approach to developing or managing clinical practice. It requires a degree of flexibility and fluidity based on firm scientific and clinical evidence validating appropriate and sustainable clinical practice.**

One of the major characteristics of evidence-based practice is the continual change in clinical practice based on the most current and relevant evidence. Any attempt at ritualizing and permanently formalizing a clinical practice simply to obtain economic advantage defeats the purpose of evidence-based methodologies. In fact, such unilateral cost-based initiatives undermine the effectiveness and value of evidence-based practice and ultimately eliminate any potential for cost saving that might be discovered in efficient and effective practice approaches.

Evidence-based practice provides a framework for a specific clinical way of life. It involves developing structures, methodologies, and clinical practice approaches that reflect a specific way of doing business. It involves a commitment in the process that is devoted to tracking down and applying the best available knowledge related to any specific clinical process, which specifically meets patient needs and answers the critical questions related to best practices. Within this paradigm, the practitioner is determined to ensure the most accurate diagnosis and treatment, and can apply the best possible information to clinical judgments related to that treatment. Evidence-based practice engages the whole range of research approaches, from randomized to the most structured, as a way of both gathering data and establishing an information base upon which to advance sound clinical decision-making (McGill, 2002).

An analogy that demonstrates the new contextual framework for the use of evidence relates to the question, "Why do physicians and nurses kill more people than airline pilots?" The answer is complex: pilots are required to have sufficient time off and complete every check in duplicate. They have sufficient checks and balances as well as redundancy in the system, follow specific and validated protocols for action, and, if committing a serious error, are required to die with their passengers. In response to this scenario, it is said that if the same rules applied to physicians, nurses, and other practitioners, there would be fewer errors and better practice in health care. Evidence-based practice begins to address this disparity, as it provides a dependable frame of reference upon which nurses, physicians, and other practitioners can depend for assessing the efficacy and effectiveness of practice and its impact on clinical outcomes (Friedland, 1998).

Currently, health care literature is impossibly diverse with a database that is unmanageably large. Furthermore, it is disorganized, uncoordinated, unwieldy, and often filled with bias. Also, much clinical research is so poorly undertaken that its validity is readily subject to question. In fact, much clinical activity is based on previous experience or clinical research that is not sufficiently accurate; it does not have a rigorous scientific design or validity to be applied to specific clinical circumstances (Bakken, Crimino, & Hripcsak, 2004). Obtaining evidence related to the large range of clinical decisions remains open to question, especially in relation to issues of number of test subjects, and the timing of testing, intervention, and treatment. Furthermore, the implications of personal mythology, sociology, psychology, and cultural concerns are frequently missing from the array of information related to appropriate and evidentiary clinical practices. All of these factors influence the clinical process and the healing dynamic, and require further explication in order to more fully understand their value and applicability.

Often, current clinical guidelines are not sufficient and do not provide the right kind of answers that clinical professionals are hoping to depend upon for clinical action and decision-making. As currently devised, they are slow to develop, require a great deal of resources of questionable generalizability, and are often surprisingly anecdotal. Taken together, it makes the current state-of-the-art with regard to clinical practice highly questionable and subject to broad variability. In this circumstance, the work of evidence-based practice is a complex yet vital undertaking that begins to more rigorously and systematically codify evidence, link experience, and create more valid and sustainable foundations for effective clinical decision-making and applied practice (Geyman, Deyo, & Ramsey, 2000).

BEGINNING WITH CRITICAL THINKING AND CLINICAL SYNTHESIS

Over the years, much has been written about reflective and critical thinking processes, especially as applied to clinical practice (Kozier, Erb Glenora, Berman, & Snyder, 2003). Critical thinking is simply the ability to deconstruct events and to reason the origins of situations (Brookfield, 1987). Essentially, critical thinking is a format or a methodology of problem solving that requires reflection and disciplined process. Critical thinking builds on particular standards, practices, protocols, values, and ideals. It is goal directed and specifically intended to inform effective decision-making. Specific characteristics unique to critical thinking include: inductive and deductive reasoning, application of knowledge; translation and interpretation of research; validation and implementation of experience; innovation and creativity; and the evaluation of impact and/or outcomes. Critical thinkers are generally systematic, organized, informed, and purposeful, such that their activities lead to defined and expected results (Oermann, 1991).

The critical thinker is able to reflect concomitantly on both information and situation. Reflected in good critical thinking are: a facility at priority setting, balancing and competing priorities; making judgments about specific risks and benefits; and the impact they might have on decision-making. The good critical thinker makes effective decisions regarding specific interventions, the timing, and subsequent decisions and their impact, and effectively communicates process, decisions, and impact to other providers and to the patient.

Critical thinkers adhere to rigorous intellectual and academic standards. As a part of this adherence, the critical thinker commits to using appropriate and referenced research information, validated and accepted data sources, as well as accurate sources for clinical decision-making. The critical thinker is always working to remain precise, clear, complete, and accurate in all decision-making and in communication. Since evidence-based practice requires the same level of rigor, there is a necessary goodness-of-fit between the demands of good critical thinking and the process expectations for evidence-based practice (Figure 1.2).

Critical reasoning, in common with the processes associated with evidence-based practice, involves the process of effective problem-solving. The critical thinker enters into the process of identifying problems and issues, and tying them as best as possible to the structure and elements of good thinking. Like evidence-based process, the critical thinker attempts to: delineate the problem;

Figure 1.2   From Process to Synthesis

From *Process* to *Synthesis*	
• **Critical Process**	• **Critical Synthesis**
• Newtonian	• Quantum
• Reductionistic	• Multi-lateral
• Provider driven	• "User driven"
• Process centric	• Value centric
• Interventional	• Referent (continuous)

understand its indications; define the elements and components of the problem; develop the frames of reference related to the problem; and, ultimately, define the direction that needs to be pursued in order to appropriately address the problem. Clearly delineating the facts of the issue and all the elements that comprise the issue helps develop a deep understanding of the basic components of the problem and drives the critical thinker toward the elements of solution seeking. The same process forms the foundation for evidence-based practice. Problem formation is the foundation for both critical thinking and the mechanics of evidence-based applications.

Evidence-based practice is purposeful and so is critical thinking. Evidence-based practice and critical thinking hold the following elements in common:

- A problem exists that requires exploration.
- There is a purpose or goal that attempts to be addressed.
- A frame of reference is constructed that looks at all of the elements of the problem.
- Assumptions about the problem, its characteristics, and elements are drawn from an assessment of the problem.
- Some central concepts, themes, and indicators emerge as a result of clarifying the problem.
- Evidence, data, information, and sources are accessed to better inform, explain, or expand the problem.
- Interpretations, evidence, applications, and protocols are informed by the aggregation of information as applied to a specific problem or situation.
- Reasoning, planning, processing, defining, and documenting lead to a format or process that will guide subsequent action in addressing the problem.
- Action consistent with the protocols and parameters is undertaken, all the while assessing process, impact, and effect.

- Mechanisms for evaluating, making judgments, adjusting, generalizing, and applying to a broader set of like problems indicate the effectiveness and utility of the critical problem-solving process (Paul, 1990).

The essential personal attributes of critical thinking and the external objective attributes of evidence-based practice combine to create the essential requisites and conditions for providing an evidence base to clinical activity. Both require an element of discipline, rigor, and objectivity to the deliberative process. Both are complementary and reflect an approach to clinical practice, the goal of which is to ensure a clear and rational basis upon which practice decisions are made and clinical activities are undertaken.

Like critical thinking, evidence-based practice requires clinical decision-makers to use the best available evidence, including clinical expertise as well as specific patient circumstances and preferences. To effectively carry out evidence-based practice, sufficient exploration, research, and evidence gathering must have been generated with regard to the specific clinical issue or case. Furthermore, the clinician must have sufficient and appropriate skills during the critical process and analysis to be able to read the research, understand its implications, translate it into the language of practice, and, finally, apply it within specific patient circumstances (Dawes, 1999).

Finally, the clinician must be able to make decisions on the evidence, implement practice, and ultimately change that practice as the evidence indicates a need for change. This fluidity and flexibility between the discipline of process and the practice, and the requisites for good outcome are cornerstones of evidence-based practice. This continual confluence between the foundations of practice and the ability to change when the need for it is articulated serves as a foundation upon which all practice parameters must be based. The challenge to historic clinical practice is found in the contradiction between the fluidity, flexibility, and commitment to changing practice when the demand for it occurs as opposed to rigid and formal policies, procedures, and practices that do not lend themselves to fluid, flexible, and immediate changes.

The processes associated with formalizing the clinical process create a challenging, yet important demand for fundamental shifts in practice. To clearly identify an issue or problem, this analysis must be based on an accurate assessment of the current knowledge base, research data, and practice. Included must be the ability and the facility to search for relevant information in the literature to glean the data upon which clear decision-making can be made. In addition, the skills necessary to evaluate the research or data generated using clearly defined criteria regarding its merit and applicability are now a fundamental aspect of clinical practice (Pape, 2003). Interventions will be chosen and will be effective to the extent that the skills necessary to undertake this process are in place in the individual practitioner and within the context of collective practice standards.

CLINICAL SYNTHESIS: EXTENDING THE NURSING PROCESS

Nursing process has been a foundation for nursing practice action for the last three decades. It is simply the nursing format for the critical thinking process. It provides a clinical overlay that is specific and unique to nursing-based activities and to achieving anticipated nursing care outcomes.

As applied to the clinical process, critical thinking has been transformed to include the elements of activity and of care. This caring component provides an overlay that is unique to the nursing experience and includes elements of interaction, relationship, communication, and satisfaction. Using formative, summative, and confirmative strategies, the critical thinking processes are transformed into nursing actions that have an impact on the patient's clinical process. These formative processes help the nurse develop understanding and create a feedback loop related specifically to personal knowledge, current applications, and the need for further learning and application of clinical care (Martin, 2002).

In the summative process, competency and the application of care become the critical centerpieces to ensure that the right choices are undertaken in the application of nursing activities, and these draw upon the nurse's critical translation skills as he or she begins to apply assessment and thought into clinical action. It is at this point that all of the critical information related to clinical action is correlated with the specific circumstances and conditions of the patient to both inform and guide critical clinical action.

The confirmative component of the critical process relates to the integration between thinking, acting, and reflecting on currency, applicability, and value of the clinical action in relationship to expectations and to clinical outcomes. Confirmation ensures that there is a relationship between the process chosen, the action undertaken, and any outcomes achieved. At this stage, the intent is to make sure that there has been a goodness-of-fit and that the expectation actually leads to changing conditions in a way that benefits the patient (Oermann, 1999).

While each of these elements is important to the active practice and application of nursing, there is a need for a shift in emphasis to reflect the characteristics of evidence construction and contemporary clinical practice. Evidence-based approaches require a heavy emphasis on the linkage and integration of information in a systematic and organized way that ultimately has an impact on choice and delivery of patient care. This notion of combining significant sources of data with appropriate decision-making and subsequent clinical activity now changes the dynamic and emphasis in clinical process. This shift changes the fundamentals of nursing process and of practice as the driving force for choice making, and subsequent action based on decisions relates to the quality and integration of the data available for good clinical decision-making.

In an era where evidence is now an essential component of validating action, becoming critical to the foundations upon which this action is taken requires that the evidence is substantial enough to justify the action and sustain it. Historically, the intensity of this relationship in clinical practice has been rather tenuous. While critical thinking and clinical process have been valuable in terms of learning and process application for nurses and other providers, what has been missing is an ability to draw on a large enough database in a way that validates the clinical choices that are subsequently made and to do so in real time. In the old model of thinking, knowledge was viewed as a capacity, that is, something that someone has and subsequently expresses, ultimately translating it into action. The flaw in this approach is the assumption that sufficient and valid knowledge is present, upon which subsequent action is taken. There is precious little evidence of the truth of this approach.

While practitioners judiciously and dutifully identify the elements of competence and build competency in clinical approaches, there is little evidence that competence is present. Ensuring competency assumes the foundations for action are clear, precise, understood, and held in common. The truth is that this rarely occurs. The only measure for adequate clinical performance that has provided any veracity is experience. Nurses and other clinicians draw heavily on the value of experience in terms of clinical activity. The problem with this, however, is that experience is based on past practice. The question related to past practice thus becomes, "What are the legitimate, clear, accurate as well as valid foundations upon which this experience is based?" Much of clinical experience is not validated by any truly objective and sustainable methodology other than the aggregation of the number of clinical processes, procedures, and clinical interventions. Without a firmer foundation driven by a continuous and dynamic access to objective and validated clinical performance, experience is just that, experience. There is no evidence, no clarity, and no validity as to whether the experience has real meaning and value. This is especially difficult in contemporary nursing, because so many nurses claim competency through valuing their own experience without recognizing that, in an evidence-based framework, such claims are more an indictment than value.

Missing most often in this scenario are the structural elements of synthesis. These include the ability to link and integrate all of the elements, sources, and databases necessary in a dynamic way to best inform decisions and action (Figure 1.2). This notion of critical clinical synthesis is now the centerpiece for clinical process in an evidence-based framework. Synthesis simply means having access to both the hardware and the software processes that are essential to make the most appropriate clinical decision under any given set of circumstances (O'Neil, Dluhy, Fortier, & Michel, 2004).

ACCESS AND CLINICAL SYNTHESIS

For evidence-based practice to be sustainable, access to a digital information framework is essential to its success. This notion of access becomes critical to the clinical process in today's framework for evidence-based practice. Access simply means the availability and ability to obtain and use information in a way that will inform practice and guide the action (Wulff & Nixon, 2004). For nurses and other clinical providers, it is the essential cornerstone of critical clinical synthesis.

This notion of clinical access skills is a fundamental cornerstone of developing both attitude and facility in evidence-based processes. An "access" clinician is one who has both facility and means to obtain real-time information in the act of clinical processing and in a way that it can be assessed, translated, applied, and evaluated within the context of the clinical circumstance. Essentially, this means that the access-enabled nurse or clinician is able to utilize real-time technology in the course of clinical decision-making and acting as a part of the process of clinical action (Podichetty & Penn, 2004a). This essential real-time approach calls for access to digital equipment and hardware as well as facility in the real-time use of software in the course of undertaking clinical work.

An evidence-based context that is fundamentally necessary for it to operate effectively over time depends upon the information and infrastructure, and its goodness-of-fit with clinical process. This real-time clinical process requires portability, fluidity, and mobility of both the hardware and software of information services in a way that increases its utility in present-time clinical decision-making and action (Hougaard, 2004). If evidence-based practice is to become a real experience for the first-line practitioner, an ongoing availability, facility, and utility of the interface between technology and clinical decision-making must become a way of life for practice. Without this integration of data and decision, evidence-based practice remains at considerable distance from reality in the lives of the majority of practitioners.

Access skill development within an evidence-based conceptual framework calls for a different approach to both basic education in clinical practice and ongoing performance expectations in the clinical environment. The education of nurses and clinicians must include higher levels of expectation with regard to development of access skills. Furthermore, it must also incorporate an understanding of the fluidity of knowledge and the development of competency in knowledge management rather than knowledge capacity (synthesis). Perhaps the greatest impediment to effective knowledge management is the prevailing notion of having enough knowledge capacity to affirm competence. It must be remembered that competency is not what one has; instead, it is what one does and the efficacy of that action. Competency is not an outcome measure; rather, it is a process value. Furthermore, competency is dynamic. It is not static, nor is it a condition that one achieves and then retains forever. Competency is fluid, reflecting currency, appropriateness, and applicability. The competency of today can become the error of tomorrow if it does not reflect the latest reality in terms of measures of effectiveness (Lucia & Lepsinger, 1999).

In addition, competency must reflect the changing dynamic of technology, information, and a state-of-the-art (or science). This fluidity of prevailing clinical reality affects the notion of competence to the extent that it cannot be contained or owned. Competency is simply a reflection of relevance, with relevance being defined as the confluence between what is the latest known information and evidence, and how relevant and related the practice that reflects it is (Dubois, 1993). That goodness-of-fit is the highest indication of competence and the best reflection of effective evidence-based practice.

Evidence-based practice calls our clinical disciplines to an entirely new approach to education for practice. Producing the competent practitioner now requires creating a skilled practitioner who is facile in computer information technology management, translation skills to apply that knowledge to the clinical situation, and a high level of real-time application and evaluation techniques that are able to both validate clinical practice and feed the outcomes of that practice back into the information loop (Horak, Welton, & Shortell, 2004). Skilled practitioners recognize the continuous, dynamic connection between the action of practice and return of information into the scientific network, so that it both informs and is informed by the action taken by individual practitioners (Eysenbach, Powell, Rizo, & Stern, 2004). This continuing dynamic between the practitioner and the virtual reality is now a fundamental element of the practice itself. Access to information, use of that information, evaluation of that information after it is applied, and feedback of that information into the database system is now a fundamental subset of the nursing process. It represents one component of the dynamic of critical synthesis.

Evidence-based practice only can be accurately and dynamically informed over time and in real-time to the extent that information can be accessed quickly, documented effectively, aggregated appropriately, and re-accessed in a continuous loop of data management, access, and application. If the nodes and networks are sufficiently complex and integrated, this dynamic can occur at the point of service, within clinical services, across organizational networks, and, conceivably, across a national database (Scavuzzo & Gamba, 2004). If best practices are ever to be truly obtained and utilized, this kind of node and network framework will necessarily become a foundation of managing clinical care nationwide.

Nodes and Networks

In evidence-based practice and in clinical synthesis, understanding the nodes and networks is critical to sustainability. Networks consist of nodes that are generally connected together by links. Networks are frequently illustrated using dots or circles that represent specific nodes, and straight and curved lines between nodes that represent the linkages (Figure 1.3). The critical element here is that the network is defined by its nodes and not by its links. Links are simply the points, lines, and processes that operate between the nodes. Nodes and networks represent real system processes and represent the theoretical framework that ultimately impacts the effective management of networks and aggregates of information. While network theory, analysis, and synthesis are a study onto themselves, it is important to recognize the impact of the network's knowledge on evidence-based practice (Moorehead & Delaney, 1998).

Network management and an awareness of the network's impact on clinical decision-making are important factors necessary to understand current time management in terms of evidence-based practice. Issues of degrees exist; for example, the numbers of direct connection to nodes indicate the kinds of connectors and hubs in the network. Elements of "betweenness," the number of direct connections in a network, help determine the degree of integration

---

Figure 1.3   Nodes and Networks

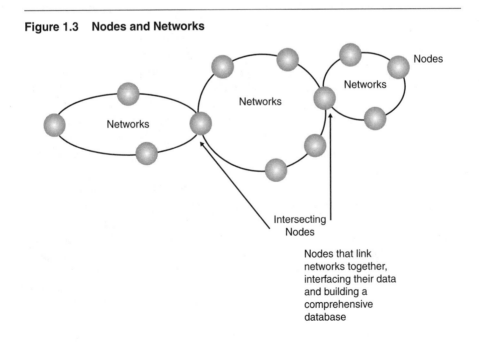

between either elements or members of the network. The degree of closeness of the nodes and the short distance between the connectors determine the level of immediacy and intensity that elements (or individuals) have in relation to each other. Those nodes that act as integrators and boundary spanners link aggregates of elements (or people) with other large data points (or groups). These major points are often entry or access points to each other, and to nodes and clusters, facilitating connection in creating the use of access to a wide radius of information. Complexity or decentralization of the network and the accommodations of the links and connections that reflect those relationships are critical influences on access and action. All of these network elements are important to the future development and management of evidence-based processes.

Understanding and applying systems management are important when constructing an infrastructure to manipulate evidence-based processes to make evidence-based practice a way of life in organizations. This calls for more than simply incremental approaches to evidence-based activities. In fact, the ability to create truly sustainable evidence-based processes requires the creation of a continuous, dynamic evidence-based infrastructure that supports, manages, and interfaces the data and practice relationship within the clinical environment, between clinical practitioners, and across specific clinical practice parameters (Saranto & Hovenga, 2004).

Here again, understanding the critical link between the digital capacity to aggregate clinical data in a pool with a huge confluence of related information, and the human ability to manage and access that network, translate it into practice, and evaluate its impact, and then feed the results back into the digital network as a cybernetic dynamic, represents the best in critical synthesis. This notion of synthesis is now a fundamental part of critical clinical practice. Nurses and other practitioners must now recognize that the ability to synthesize a broad diversity of information, circumstances, conditions, and patient vagaries in a way that influences critical judgment and subsequent clinical action is the foundation to contemporary practice.

Critical synthesis calls for the practitioner—primarily the nurse—to be able to live at the intersection and recognize that the practitioner is essentially managing the intersection and addressing the confluence of elements and forces operating there, linking them and using them in a way that has a positive impact on patient care (Segal, Dunt, & Day, 2004). Living at the intersection, which includes managing the variables that define clinical life, making decisions, and undertaking clinical practices, is the focal point of contemporary and future clinical practice. Competency, in this set of circumstances, is reflected in the ability to manage this confluence of factors and forces, integrate them, prioritize them, make decisions, and, finally, act. This is nursing synthesis.

Evidence-based practice draws on an increasing level of understanding related to systems processes and their application to clinical decision-making. A systematic day-to-day management of information, digital infrastructure, and clinical practice is essential for administrative and management leadership in creating a supportive environment for evidence-based practice. This new environment further requires a shift in the mental model of organizational structure and human systems. The movement from a 20th century model of finite institutional structural references is giving way to more fluid, flexible, portable, and mobile notions of structure and organizational format (Porter-O'Grady, Hawkins, & Parker, 1997). Furthermore, health care leaders have to reconceptualize the organizational structure of clinical services and practice environments. As the information infrastructure, the Internet, and other digital and fiber-optic infrastructures become a common context for social and clinical life, leaders must reconceive the organization and system structures that support it. Perhaps the greatest impediment to the success of evidence-based practice is the organizational, informational, and interactional infrastructure necessary to support it. Without these structures of support, format, and infrastructure, it will be impossible to sustain an evidence-based frame of reference for ongoing clinical practice into the future (Figure 1.4).

BUILDING THE INFORMATION INFRASTRUCTURE FOR EVIDENCE-BASED PRACTICE

If we are to ensure that evidence-based practice does not become another fad in health care, it is important to build a systematic organizational infrastructure that supports this method as a way of delivering care. From the information in-

Figure 1.4   New Model of 21st Century Practice

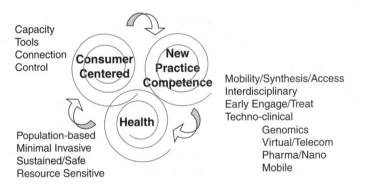

Capacity
Tools
Connection
Control

Consumer Centered

New Practice Competence

Health

Mobility/Synthesis/Access
Interdisciplinary
Early Engage/Treat
Techno-clinical
   Genomics
   Virtual/Telecom
   Pharma/Nano
   Mobile

Population-based
Minimal Invasive
Sustained/Safe
Resource Sensitive

frastructure to the interdisciplinary and organizational framework, new approaches to organizing and delivering care are essential.

Creating an Interdisciplinary Frame of Reference

Perhaps the most difficult and challenging aspects of contemporary clinical practice within an evidence-based framework are the traditional compartmentalization and fragmentation of disciplinary practice (Coombs & Ersser, 2004). Historically, the disciplines, especially nursing and medicine, have developed on parallel but distinct pathways. In an effort to establish independent professional and economic frames for practice, nursing and medicine have remained essentially nonaligned. As the complexity of health care has increased and the intensity of clinical practice within disciplines has accelerated, the relationships between them have become even more distinct, perhaps even polarized (LeTourneau, 2004). What is unusual about this set of circumstances at this time of clinical and technical integration is that the behavior patterns of independence are no longer relevant to the clinical necessity for integration.

The highly independent practice of medicine and the equally complex interdependent practice of nursing now must intersect in a highly interrelated format if evidence-based practice is to be sustained. Furthermore, this clinical intersection between the two major disciplines must also include a concomitant and equally important multidisciplinary intersection between all key disciplines. This will not happen by accident. Clinical leadership in health care must construct the format for integration and interaction necessary to create the structural and organizational foundations that support interdisciplinary evidence-based practices. Critical among those efforts are:

- Each discipline must clearly define its specific and unique accountability for clinical decision-making, clinical action, and interdisciplinary interaction.
- A mandate and organizational format must require the disciplines to develop clinical protocols and practices in conjunction with each other, such that no discipline unilaterally develops clinical practices that impact other disciplines.
- A structural format must require the decision-making processes of each discipline to act in concert, such that no one discipline can make clinical decisions in isolation of its relationship to other disciplines.
- A clearly defined process, methodology, or mechanism for constructing clinical protocols is ongoing business between the disciplines, and within the process of making decisions that conform to clinical protocols and formats.

- A clinical management structure needs to reflect particular interdisciplinary configurations based on specified organizational formats that support effective interdisciplinary clinical decision-making, activities, and evaluation.

Systematic approaches to organizing and structuring the disciplines are important to systematic delineation and evaluation of care. In fact, evidence-based practice requires an organizing format that essentially forces the disciplines to integrate their clinical activities, reflecting an essential synthesis or confluence of clinical process related to patient care and effective practice. The challenge to creating and sustaining a structural format relates specifically to the past independence and nonaligned practice relationships established by the disciplines independent of each other. Historic disciplinary, gender, knowledge, legal, legislative, and relational issues are clearly in the first line of dialogue. Much of the cultural and organizational shifts that need to occur are reflected in how these historic issues are resolved, and how subsequent action represents a new set of relationships around these long-held practices.

Getting Past Cultural and Organizational Barriers

Evidence-based practice therefore has cultural and organizational implications that are vital to its success. Evidence-based practice will remain a marginal or faddish practice if the interdisciplinary interface necessary to advance it does not become a central component of its implementation. When examining organizational mandates, managers and clinical leaders need to realize that the structure for integrated, corollary, and horizontal relationships will be as important as the clinical processes related to establishing evidence in practice. Several priorities must emerge within the manager's table of accountability if the organizational structure supporting evidence-based practice is to operate effectively:

- Create a leadership lexicon that represents the collaborating, correlating, and horizontal relationship between the disciplines and management processes associated with it.
- Create an organizational structure that creates equity, collaboration, dialogue, and distributed decision-making frames of reference for the function and operation of clinically specific services.
- Move away from the organizational delineation of clinical services based on models of medical diagnosis rather than processes of patient care.
- Eliminate turf-based clinical service structures that create discipline-specific clinical alignments and subordinate other disciplines within those

alignments, which reflects a change from a pyramidal orientation of authority to more circular clinical relationships and decision-making.

- End the "captain of the ship" mental model for organizational and relational
  interaction between the disciplines, recognizing instead a complexity-based,
  collaborative decision model for patient care.
- Move to end hierarchy-based pyramidal models of control and decision authority, replacing them with point-of-service oriented clinical decision formats driven by patient care professionals.
- Enhance the skills of the management and clinical leadership team to
  include more facilitative, engaged, and clinically driven decision processes
  and empowerment strategies to more fully engage practitioners in continuous evidence-based practices.

Clearly, new organizational arrangements to create a different set of parameters for practitioners are essential to build the organizational frame necessary to make evidence-based practice a fundamental system of doing business in
health care. Managers must understand that the prevailing organizational models of decision-making, organizing, and structuring relationships are impediments
to engaging practitioners more fully in decisions about effective practice. After
years of parental and hierarchical organizational constructs in health care driven
by lay business models of organizing work, the evidence is overwhelming that
clinical practice and quality patient care are sacrificed to a high degree in such
models. What is important is that sound business principles be applied to clinical service structures. Equally important is that the outcomes of clinical practice
not be lost in the effort to maintain financial viability. Loss of focus on the core
business end of health care and failure to facilitate cost-effective, outcome oriented, and sustainable clinical practice ultimately results in the loss of the financial viability of the health care organization.

If evidence-based principles are to be applied effectively in the clinical framework of the health care system, they must be applied equally effectively in the
management and organizational framework. Evidence-based practice does not
only mean clinical activity. The mental model for evidence must permeate the
organization and every level of its structure. Clinical efficacy and effectiveness
simply should be the results of structural integrity, good financial stewardship,
and excellent patient care. Interface between each of these is as important as the
effectiveness of any one of them. Evidence-based practice in the clinical frame
of reference is no more sustainable than it would be if operated only in the financial constructs of the organization. Indeed, the true viability of evidence-
based practice is found in the intersection of all of the organizational, systematic,
and clinical variables affecting the delivery of high quality patient care. Indeed,
the measurement of each of these in relationship to the other is the best exam-

ple of an evidence-based practice framework for clinical services. As a result, in the interface between structural, business, and clinical activities, leaders must recognize the continuing and intersecting dynamics essential to maintain focus on the core business and for sustaining excellence at all levels of measurement (Figure 1.5).

Just as necessary in the information infrastructure, the organizational structure must sacrifice the historic addiction to hierarchical control, replacing it with a commitment to a highly effective and strongly delineated valuing of horizontal relationship, accountability, individual and collective performance, and evidence of sustainable levels of measurable quality clinical service (Coombs, 2003). Equally important is that management's demands for accountability, performance-based decision-making, professional and individual evaluation, and clinical expectations and outcomes are correlated in a way that demonstrates a confluence of these factors on maintaining high levels of patient care and of organizational excellence. Here again, the interface between the information infrastructure, performance measurement, and quality patient care is critical. Evidence-based outcomes cannot be obtained simply through the definition of clinical protocols and the clarity around the clinical expectations. Without clearly defined relationships between competence, performance, expectations, and outcomes, there would be a superficial and slippery foundation upon which evidence-based practices would be built.

Perhaps the greatest problem with current notions of evidence-based practice is the belief that simply getting at the practices by identifying the relationship to expectations and outcomes will be sufficient to ultimately improve

Figure 1.5   Building Clinical Evidence

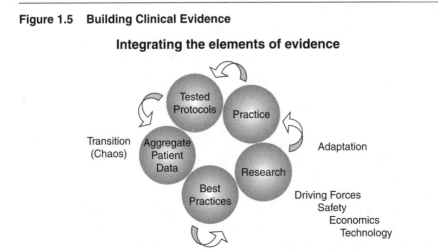

Integrating the elements of evidence

patient care, reduce risk, and advance the practice of medicine. Nothing could be further from the truth. This synthetic and superficial notion of what is necessary to sustain evidence-based practice will surely contribute to its decline. Managers and clinical leaders must reflect on their understanding and in the design of organizations, the fundamental interface between organizational structure, performance expectations, clinical protocols and practices, and evaluation of clinical care as an outcome of the intersection between all of these variables.

This understanding, of course, should exclude no discipline. This notion of the medical staff as customers of the organization rather than as partners in practice is a key impediment to obtaining the kind of medical accountability that is critical to effective evidence-based practice. No disciplines can remain outside the cycle of accountability and expect that practice will be enhanced or improved. Expressing and owning accountability for fiscal, relational, interactional, and disciplinary contribution to defining clinical protocols and practice behavior are essential to success and must include all involved disciplines. Neither employment nor partnership is an effective excluding consideration.

While most physicians in the American health care system are not employed, they have a history of directing decisions that affect what those who are employed in hospitals and health care systems do. This "closed shop" approach to medical practice is no longer viable nor is it sustainable, especially within the construct of evidence-based practice. The "physician as customer" notion must dissipate from the language of administrators and managers in health care. It must be replaced by the language of partnership and accountability. Evidence-based practice requires a level of equity and collaborative expectations of all those addressed under its rubric. The physician continues to be a key player in this clinical drama. While the complexities of health care and increased intensity of investment and involvement of all the disciplines have created an interdependence that simply cannot be dissolved, the physician often remains the point of access. No longer can physicians remain outside the circular cycle of relationships necessary to identify protocols, methodologies, practices, and evaluation of the clinical activities that are reflective of the intersections and the intensity of the multiplicity of clinical providers making decisions along the patient's clinical pathway. Just as in the information infrastructure, access to each other as clinical partners is critical to both the developmental and application elements of evidence-based practice. Access to each other's practice, data, protocols, and clinical behaviors is essential when seeking the normative as well as the path to excellence. Mythology and ignorance of each other's action and contribution to decision-making and clinical practice are no longer viable in rendering a clearly delineated and validated level of clinical care (Thomas, Sexton, & Helmreich, 2003).

For clinical leaders and managers, much of the initial effort in building the infrastructure for evidence-based practice is in reconstructing the formal organizational as well as professional and personal relationships within the clinical service. This requires thinking and acting in fundamentally different ways with regard to the role of the leader in formatting support systems for evidence-based clinical services. Predominant in the leader's armamentarium are the following elements:

- An ability to facilitate interdisciplinary dialogue from the simple to the complex with the intention of establishing the continuing and sustainable mode of communication between disciplines
- Gathering diverse stakeholders together around controversial and "noisy" issues with an ability to achieve an agreeable outcome for all stakeholders
- Helping others delineate clear performance expectations as well as individual and collective accountability for performance, holding each to the commitments and tasks agreed upon
- Developing mechanisms and modalities of organizational and systems support for the clinical decisions and subsequent actions made by the disciplines in advancing patient care
- Addressing crisis, nonperformance, and conflict as a normal part of the managerial function, with the intent of seeking common ground and facilitating sustainable resolution

Leadership is no easy task. This is certainly no less so in an environment that promulgates and facilitates an evidence-based framework for clinical practice. It is vital to the success of evidence-based practice processes that the organization be fully committed to establishing evidence as a frame of reference at all levels of doing business. Consistency and faithfulness to this commitment are essential leadership and administrative criteria upon which the success of evidence-based practice can be predicated. Like most clinical processes, evidence-based practice is sustained on the altar of effective administrative support, continuous organizational encouragement and expectation, and the effective application of leadership skills. Concepts like evidence-based practice rarely fail because the concept is not viable. They often fail because the organization's priorities and leadership skills do not interface well with the expectations and demands for change in personal and organizational behavior necessary to support it.

Organizational leadership is often averse to risk and organizational noise. This fear of organizational reaction (especially within the physician community) frequently creates retrenchment and often detours the organization's leadership from the focus that must be maintained through the challenging and high decibel periods of organizational change (Lancaster, 1998). This reality is no less true with evidence-based practice when perceived as a systems change. The dramatic shift in locus of control, accountability, expectations, performance, and measurement truly creates significant organizational and systematic noise. A good administrator/manager must anticipate this prior to the organization's commitment to effective patient care and evidence-based practices. This anticipation should lead to good preparation, skill development, and careful execution of the supporting and application processes necessary to ensure effective evidence-based practice approaches.

Wise leaders do not enter the arena of evidence-based practice either incrementally or tentatively. Evidence-based practice signifies an entirely new approach to the delivery of high-quality and effective patient care. It incorporates all that is known about what works and what doesn't work. It also begins to utilize a high level of intensity of all data that are now available in the digital management of patient care. The leader understands that evidence-based practice reflects the incorporation of a completely new range of processes and elements of data, decision-making, and clinical action. The leader sees this interface between the emerging systems of complexity, digital processes, accountability, and expectations for performance and high quality outcomes as a frame of reference for the future of health care practice (Paquette, 2003). Recognizing this as a frame of reference for the future of health care, this leader sees evidence-based practice as the format for a business lifestyle in this contemporary age and for moving the professions, organizations, patients, and the social system into a 21st century framework for the delivery of health care services, which advances the quality of care and raises the level of health.

INFORMATION INFRASTRUCTURE SUPPORTING EVIDENCE-BASED PRACTICE

Evidence-based practice requires a level of information integrity and integration not achieved before in the practice environment of health care. While it is certainly true that incremental evidence-based activities can use a fairly basic array of data steps, establishing a systematic and broad-based approach to building an evidence-based framework requires a much more sophisticated integration between clinical practice and data management.

To build an information foundation and effective clinical data management, the critical factor is access. Basic clinical information availability is only one element of access assessment, however. A systematic approach to access means that the evidence-based organization has an information and operational infrastructure that provides broad-based data access to all available clinical resources in real-time, at the point of service to clinical practitioners. This level of sophistication calls for an organizational commitment to building a clinically based information infrastructure that is not yet evident in most health care institutions across the country. The primary fear about relationships in sustainable evidence-based practice today relates to the willingness of clinical organizations to make the financial, resource, and organizational commitments to building a well-designed, practitioner-friendly clinical information management system. In evidence-based practice, there must be a mechanism for integrating existing and historic clinical data, historic and current patient information as well as existing clinical practice standards and processes, and linking these individual databases together in a comprehensive, integrated data framework to guide clinical decision-making (Figure 1.6).

Databases must be able to be accessed simultaneously and in real-time. The clinician has to have the ability to act on a relatively seamless intersection of data in a way in which judgments can be made and practice actions can be undertaken. Furthermore, the clinician must be able to record instantaneously both the action and impact of clinical practices based on the data mining that occurred in making the choices for the most appropriate clinical action. Here again, evidence-based practice must be seen as a practice process, not an evaluation mechanism. Evidence-based practice must be designed and developed in an organization as a way of delivering care and a method of doing the clinical business of the organization. Therefore, data management and clinical processing must be directly related in such a way that both are ongoing elements and a subset of the full definition of clinical care (Nada, Keravnou, & Blaz, 1997).

Designing practice within an evidence-based format calls for focus on the following key elements:

- A digital documentation system that includes the digital patient records, digital hardware, portability/mobility-based recording and documentation, and software, which facilitates integration of diffuse clinical information
- Hardware that allows multiple points of access to the same patients and clinical information for a variety of involved health care professionals
- Software ensuring continuous real-time access to the multitude of collateral clinical information provided by any practitioner at every moment in the patient care continuum
- Implications of specific clinical data in relationship to other elements of clinical data must be highlighted in a way that indicate anomalies or abnormalities in real-time and available to all clinicians
- Design of the information infrastructure to accommodate the aggregation of evaluative data in ways that automatically enumerate the norms of practice with particular patients, clinical protocols, and/or practices, and subsequently informing standards of patient care

Figure 1.6 Evidence-based Clinical System

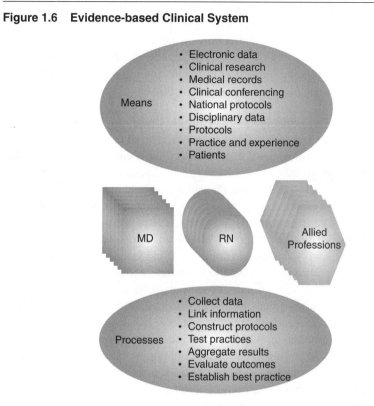

Constructing this infrastructure calls for a level of understanding the multiplicity of interfaces that are necessary to ensure that the data management process is effective. Several levels of construction are important to ensure that the right data infrastructure is available within the health care facility. Several levels of delineation are important here:

1. Specific clinical protocols are developed with regard to the predominant patient care populations, diagnosis-related groups (DRGs), or specific clinical delineation.
2. Interdisciplinary integration of clinical standards of practice are developed and linked within particular patient care populations, DRGs, or specific clinical delineation.
3. Standards of practice are agreed upon by all the disciplines and become the format for clinical decision-making action as well as clinical and patient evaluation.

4. Adjustments of clinical practice can be made in real-time as clinical performance, patient response, and immediate clinical measurement indicate a need for change in specific clinical practice.
5. Individual applications of clinical protocols/standards can be aggregated with the larger consolidated patient database as a mechanism for further validating, refining, adjusting, or validating particular clinical approaches.

Clinical design professionals recognize that two concomitant processes are occurring. The first process relates specifically to the development of clinical protocols and frames of reference for practice to provide the evidence foundation for particular clinical standards and practices. Simultaneously, the evidence-based practice format calls for real-time decisions, applications, and adjustments that are practice-based established protocols, which also reflect adjustments in patient circumstances and conditions. The information infrastructure provides a vehicle to link the developed protocol with the real-time decision-making, action, documentation, and evaluation. In addition, clinical adjustments, variances, corrective action, or standards enhancements must be available sufficiently to affect subsequent practices and/or specific populations across the clinical service spectrum. In short, these changes and adjustments that ultimately result in a shift in the protocol or standard must be available to all practitioners immediately in order for the value of evidence to impact the action of practice. It is this ongoing, living interface between the establishment of sound practice protocols based on the last available data and clinical process and real-time clinical activity and its impact that ensures the effectiveness and ongoing utility of evidence-based practice.

In establishing the foundations of evidence-based practice, availability of data becomes critical. Multifile indices of discipline-specific scientific journals (especially those on the Internet, that is, e-journals) must be easily and generally accessible. Clinically sound studies that report accurate, meaningful research have been conducted using evidence-based methodologies found using OVID or Medline key word searches. The information structure and the clinical skills necessary to access these resources must be in place in order to guide utility. Many e-guidelines and databases are merging on the worldwide Web that can provide both data and format guidance to those who are constructing or using evidence-based approaches (Bennett, Casebeer, Kristofco, & Strasser, 2004).

Simply building access to clinical information is not sufficient to ensure that it is appropriate and utilized. To date, the evidence-based practice approach has failed to really show that there has been adequate translation of best practices into appropriate clinical protocols and with standard practices within the organization. Of course, there are many behavioral, structural, and organizational reasons for this observation (Podichetty & Penn, 2004b). Perhaps the most significant factor is that much of evidence-based practice remains discipline unilateral and clinically nonaligned. Knowledge is good, but unless it is aggregated, linked, and ultimately translated into continuous behavior, it is not effective.

Clinical interventions that reflect the assessment and management of the potential barriers in multidisciplinary activities can often be more effective than simply addressing the clinical protocols themselves. First, identifying those cross-discipline standards of practice and protocols upon which all disciplines agree can provide a firmer foundation for building evidence-based practice than simply incorporating other disciplines' recommendations and advice into a particular discipline-specific set of standards. Establishing this approach as a principal standard helps inform and define the clinical standards and protocols to which ultimately all will adhere. Designing the systems infrastructures to incorporate this as a principle of design builds the format for interdisciplinary collaboration and integration that becomes the prevailing characteristic of a systematic evidence-based practice approach.

CREATING A CULTURE OF EVIDENCE

This is a new world for clinical practice. As practitioners enter more fully into the digital age, the mechanisms upon which they once depended for clinical decision-making, practice application, and documentation are quickly passing. The manual and mechanical processes for critical thinking, acting, documenting, and evaluating are no longer valid in an increasingly digital world. This understanding of the virtual implications intersecting the course of human life is in stark contrast to the process-driven clinical orientation still evident in most practitioners today.

The challenge for clinical leaders in this set of circumstances is to not simply introduce a framework for evidence-based practice. Instead, it is the transformation of the entire approach to health care delivery. A deep understanding that most health care reflects a provider-driven model of clinical decision-making and acting that is bereft of ownership and accountability for health is important to the demand for undertaking major shifts in health care delivery. Leadership must be able to see a need for change to support evidence-based practice at three levels of intensity: systems change, disciplinary change, and individual change. This chapter has enumerated some of the fundamental concepts that are essential to those meaningful long-term changes necessary to support evidence-based practice as a way of undertaking clinical work in the 21st century. Initiation of evidence-based practice can occur in a number of simple, functional steps that are outlined in a variety of ways in subsequent chapters. It is important to keep in mind that, to make evidence-based practice tenable in the context of our digital age, a radical transformation in all the elements of practice is essential to sustain it and to make a positive difference in the lives of patients.

Even more important to the delivery of effective quality health care is the commitment of every individual practitioner in making evidence-based practice the format and framework for individual decision-making and clinical activity. Every practitioner needs to address fundamental and specific conditions in order to ensure appropriate and effective patient care. Some priorities include:

- An individual critical review of current practice behaviors and dependencies upon which past practice has been based that are an impediment to the engagement of emerging practice requisites
- Development of a thorough and clear understanding of the elements of evidence-based practice and the implications they have for personal and professional practice, interdisciplinary relationships, and effective patient care
- Full engagement of each practitioner and every discipline to communicate and interact with each other in a common effort to effectively define individual and collective contributions to clinical protocols and practice as an ongoing way of undertaking patient care
- An individual professional commitment to continually evaluate the action of practice, subjecting it to the test of analysis and comparison for the purposes of improving and advancing practice
- A personal, sustaining commitment to a continuously changing practice that is no longer absolutely defined by ritual and routine, which ultimately represents the best response to evidence and outcome
- A commitment on the part of every practicing professional to engage with her or his colleagues in a collective exercise to more clearly define the foundations of practice, joining with other disciplines and with patients to define the foundations of practice, change the elements of practice, advance positive clinical outcomes, and raise the level of social health.

In the final analysis, if evidence-based practice is to work and be sustained, it requires commitment at every level of the health system. From government and the private sector to corporate and community health systems, to professions and providers as well as patients and communities, each will be required to participate in a fundamental change in the foundations of health care delivery. Evidence-based practice provides a format and means for creating effective change in the way health care is delivered and in the subsequent higher value obtained from health service providers.

Ultimately, the commitment to improving and changing practice must, at some level, relate to the improvements of the health of society at the individual and collective levels. Reducing errors, establishing practice foundations, and advancing quality are all important elements of effective health care delivery systems. However, the more important measure of health care delivery is the quality of health of the citizens of the community and of the nation. Evidence-based practice must, in the long run, have a definitive impact. In a critical time in American history, indeed, human history, focusing on the quality of health for all has become increasingly important as we move more inevitably to becoming a global community. As the tenure of life is extended by the miracle of technology and our social constructs continually demand reconfiguration, movements of the health care system into a new frame of reference will be important to its long-term viability. The use of the information infrastructure, emerging digital, nano, and mobility-based technologies will further refine and raise the level of impact that health care therapeutics will have on the future of health. As portable therapeutics become a greater component of the delineation and maintenance of the health of an aging population, the clinical, social, economic, and personal impacts will be significant. The age of evidence is truly an age of engagement and validation, a way of delineating the value of decisions, actions, and outcomes. Evidence-based practice provides a means, and perhaps a foundation, upon which 21st century health care will be built. Recognizing the significance of the work, the depth of the activities associated with building mechanisms for evidence, and the commitment necessary to sustain and advance a new framework for health care delivery is the most important clinical work of our time.

REFERENCES

Bakken, S., Crimino, J., & Hripcsak, G. (2004). Promoting patient safety and enabling evidenced based practice through informatics. *Medical Care, 42*(2), 49–56.

Bennett, N., Casebeer, L., Kristofco, R., & Strasser, S. (2004). Positions Internet information seeking behavior. *Journal of Continuing Education in the Health Professions, 24*(1), 31–38.

Breslin, E., & Lucas, V. (2003). *Women's Health Nursing: Towards Evidence Based Practice.* Chicago: W. B. Saunders.

Brookfield, S. (1987). *Developing Critical Thinkers: Challenging Adults to Explore Alternative Ways of Thinking and Acting.* Milton Keynes, UK: Open University Press.

Coombs, M. (2003). Power and conflict in intensive care clinical decision-making. *Intensive & Critical Care Nursing, 19*(3), 125–135.

Coombs, M., & Ersser, S. (2004). Medical hegemony in decision-making—a barrier to interdisciplinary working in intensive care? *Journal of Advanced Nursing, 46*(3), 245–252.

Dawes, M. (1999). *Evidence Based Practice: A Primer for Healthcare Professionals.* London, UK: Churchill Livingstone.

Dubois, D. (1993). *Competency-Based Performance Improvement: A Strategy for Organizational Change.* Amherst, MA: HRD Press.

Eysenbach, G., Powell, J., Rizo, C., & Stern, A. (2004). Health-related virtual communities and electronic support groups: Systematic review of the effects of online peer-to-peer interactions. *British Medical Journal, 328*(7449), 1166–1176.

Friedland, D. (1998). *Evidence Based Medicine: A Framework for Clinical Practice.* New York: McGraw-Hill.

Geyman, J., Deyo, R., & Ramsey, S. (2000). *Evidence Based Clinical Practice: Concepts and Approaches.* London, UK: Butterworth-Heinemann.

Horak, B., Welton, W., & Shortell, S. (2004). Crossing the quality chasm: Implications for health services administration education. *Journal of Health Administration Education, 21*(1), 15–38.

Hougaard, J. (2004). Developing evidence based interdisciplinary care standards and implications for improving patient safety. *International Journal of Medical Informatics, 73*(7/8), 615–624.

Kozier, B., Erb, G., Berman, A., & Snyder, S. (2003). *Fundamentals of Nursing Concepts: Process and Practice.* New York: Prentice Hall.

Lancaster, J. (1998). *Nursing Issues in Leading in Managing Change.* St. Louis, MO: C. V. Mosby.

Law, M. (2002). *Evidence-Based Rehabilitation: A Guide to Practice.* New York: Delmar Learning.

LeTourneau, B. (2004). Physicians and nurses: Friends or focus? *Journal of Healthcare Management, 49*(1), 12–15.

Lucia, A., & Lepsinger, R. (1999). *Art and Science of Competency Models: Pinpointing Critical Success Factors in Organizations.* San Francisco: Jossey-Bass.

Martin, C. (2002). The theory of critical thinking in nursing. *Nursing Education Perspectives, 23*(6), 243–247.

Mazurek, B., Melnyk, E., & Fineout-Overholt, E. (2004). *Evidence Based Practice in Nursing and Healthcare: A Guide to Best Practice.* Philadelphia: Lippincott, Williams & Wilkins.

McGill, S. (2002). Evidenced based prevention and rehabilitation. In *Low Back Disorders.* San Francisco: Human Kinetics Publishing.

Moorehead, S., & Delaney, C. (1998). *Information Systems Innovations for Nursing: New Vision's Adventures.* New York: Sage.

Muir, G. (2001). *Evidence Based Healthcare.* Chicago: W. B. Saunders.

Nada, L., Keravnou, E., & Blaz, Z. (1997). *Intelligent Data Analysis in Medicine and Pharmacology.* New York: Kluwer Academic Publishers.

O'Neil, E., Dluhy, N., Fortier, P., & Michel, H. (2004). Knowledge acquisition, synthesis and validation: A model for decision support systems. *Journal of Advanced Nursing, 47*(2), 134–142.

Oermann, M. (1991). *Professional Nursing Practice: A Conceptual Approach.* Philadelphia: Lippincott, Williams & Wilkins.

Oermann, M. (1999). Critical thinking, critical practice. *Nursing Management, 30*(4), 40–45.

Pape, T. (2003). Evidence based nursing practice: To infinity and beyond. *Journal of Continuing Education in Nursing, 34*(4), 189–190.

Paquette, L. (2003). *Prescription for Change: Managing and Controlling Change in Health Services.* Hauppauge, NY: Nova Science Publishers.

Paul, R. (1990). *Critical Thinking: What Every Person Needs to Survive in a Rapidly Changing World.* Rohnert Park, CA: Center for Critical Thinking and Moral Critique.

Podichetty, V., & Penn, D. (2004a). The progress of roles of electronic medicine: Benefits, concerns, and costs. *American Journal of the Medical Sciences of the Medical Sciences, 328*(2), 94–109.

Podichetty, V., & Penn, D. (2004b). The progressive roles of electronic medicine: Benefits, concerns, and costs. *American Journal of the Medical Sciences, 328*(2), 94–109.

Porter-O'Grady, T., Hawkins, M., & Parker, M. (1997). *Whole Systems Shared Governance: Architecture for Integration.* Boston: Jones and Bartlett Publishers.

Porter-O'Grady, T., & Malloch, K. (2003). *Quantum Leadership: A Textbook of New Leadership.* Boston: Jones and Bartlett Publishers.

Sackett, D., Straus, S., Richardson, S., Rosenberg, W., & Haynes, B. (2000). *Evidence-Based Medicine: How to Practice and Teach EBM.* London, UK: Churchill Livingstone.

Saranto, K., & Hovenga, E. (2004). Information literacy—what is it about? Literature review of the concept and the context. *International Journal of Medical Informatics, 73*(6), 503–513.

Scavuzzo, J., & Gamba, N. (2004). Bridging the gap: The virtual chemotherapy unit. *Journal of Pediatric Oncology Nursing, 21*(1), 27–32.

Segal, L., Dunt, D., & Day, S. (2004). Introducing coordinated care: Evaluation of design features and implementation processes implications for preferred health system model. *Health Policy, 69*(2), 215–228.

Thomas, E., Sexton, J., & Helmreich, R. (2003). Discrepant attitudes about teamwork among critical care nurses and physicians. *Critical Care Medicine, 31*(3), 956–962.

Wulff, J., & Nixon, N. (2004). Quality markers and the use of electronic journals in an academic health sciences library. *Journal of the Medical Library Association, 92*(3), 315–322.

CHAPTER 2

A Framework for Nursing Clinical Inquiry: Pathway Toward Evidence-Based Nursing Practice

Dolora C. Sanares, and Diane Heliker

Knowledge cannot be inherited or bequeathed. Knowledge rapidly becomes obsolete, so it has to be acquired anew by every individual (Drucker, 2002). Disciplined Clinical Inquiry (DCI) provides nurses an opportunity to learn and engage in "knowledge work" in nontraditional ways. These challenges and opportunities are available to every professional nurse and provide pathways to embrace the journey of nursing with enthusiasm and anticipation. Beginning with Florence Nightingale, nurses have always been encouraged to commit themselves to lifelong learning as a part of practice. If this indeed becomes the credo and practice ethic of every one of us, then practice that is based on the *best evidence* comes as a natural outgrowth.

DCI is a paradigmatic shift in achieving the joint optimization of interdisciplinary goals and values of health care providers within the framework of their respective professional philosophy and organizational mission. The DCI process brings together an integrated caring community of health professionals and patients. Implementation of DCI has introduced clinical nurses to a new practice ethic. These nurses are making a difference, the depth and breadth of which is limited only by their own motivation and desire for improving the quality of their practice. Once DCI immersion is experienced by an optimum number of clinical nurses, this practice ethic evolves and eventually becomes the normative culture, laying the cornerstone of a caring environment for clinical nurses and the patients they serve.

Beyond institutional boundaries, DCI represents a cutting-edge paradigm that redefines the value and essence of an accountable nursing practice so critical in meeting the current requirements and challenges of health care for the future. Individual and collective contributions of nurses will be the repository of knowledge recognized and applied across the clinical enterprise. Nurses choose to practice and remain engaged in practice arenas that support this culture.

Consequently, it is within these settings that patients will choose to entrust their care, to restore and achieve optimal health and wellness.

This chapter describes the framework and implementation of a model, DCI, which provides a pathway toward evidence-based nursing practice (EBNP). The theoretical underpinnings of this model, critical social theory (Friere, 1970; Habermas, 1987; Lewin, 1946), are articulated along with the methodology, participatory action research (Stringer, 1996; Stringer & Genat, 2004), used to develop each of the phases. The uniqueness of DCI is its flexibility and utility as an evidence-based practice (EBP) guide for all nurses and across all settings. DCI's user-friendly format is adaptable to all specialties and situations. The objectives of this chapter are to: (a) describe the assumptions and phases of DCI and its relevance to EBNP; and (b) provide a blueprint for the reader who may wish to incorporate DCI in a particular setting.

DCI has been inductively developed using the shared visions and experiences of nurses who voiced their interests and perceived educational needs as they participated in every phase of the pilot process. Discussion of changes, challenges, and opportunities within the current and emerging health care environment in Chapter 1 provides the context and significance that call for a collaborative and pragmatic approach to clinical inquiry and knowledge development in all health care settings. DCI offers that approach.

INCREASING AWARENESS AND OPENNESS TO CHANGE

Am I providing the highest possible level of safe, quality, and cost-effective patient-centered care? Do my current strategies for updating my practice, acquiring evidence-based information and knowledge, and developing state-of-the-art clinical skills enable me to meet the growing complexity and changing needs and demands of my patient population? These questions inspired a group of frontline nurses and managers to come to recognize that new approaches and portable tools that function in a dynamic environment would raise the standard of practice. This new approach of clinical inquiry had to be practical and applicable for each situation. Therefore, emphasis had to be placed on the local context and local expertise of the practicing nurse. This strategy had to address the long-standing gap between theoretical generalizations and specific patient interventions.

Nurses have always acknowledged the uniqueness of each patient and are aware of their clinical wisdom (Benner, 1999, 2000). The value of this wisdom and best evidence, meaning all the ways of knowing that nurses use as they come to understand patients' specific concerns, inspires nurses to devise realistic solutions in relationships with patients and families while practicing in high intensity and complex situations. The voices of all health care stakeholders had to be equally valued. This approach would ensure a sense of community and shared ownership in developing a new practice ethic and a culture of quality care. This all-inclusive culture would include nurses, managers, administrators, patients, and families, as well as members of other disciplines. Partnerships with faculty in the academic school of nursing would further increase levels of support and expertise. DCI represents such an approach.

EVIDENCE-BASED NURSING PRACTICE

In the past, clinical decisions relied on clinical experience, expert opinion, collegial relationships, pathophysiology, common sense, community standards, published materials, and other sources. The process of EBP uses the same sources of clinical advice, but passes all of them through the filter of the question, On what evidence is the advice based (Berg, 2000, p. 25)? Within the framework of the DCI model, EBNP emphasizes clinical decision-making based on the integration of the most current available best evidence. Sources of this evidence that can best inform nursing practice within this framework include: research, clinical expertise, patient's values (Sackett, Straus, Richardson, Rosenberg, & Haynes, 2000) and perspectives, and other recognized sources of knowledge (e.g., ethical knowing, socio-political knowing, personal experience, and aesthetic ways of knowing) (Carper, 1978; Silva, Sorrell, & Sorrell, 1995; White, 1995).

Guided by a focused question, it is helpful to first access nationally recognized clinical practice guidelines. Clinical practice guidelines have been referred to as systematically developed statements derived from the most current available best evidence that provide direction to practitioners in deciding among appropriate health care options for a specific clinical condition. In the United States, the National Guideline Clearinghouse (NGC; Web site, http://www.guideline.gov/) is an Internet-based public resource that provides a comprehensive database of evidence-based clinical practice guidelines and related documents. NGC is supported by the Agency for Healthcare Research and Quality, U.S. Department of Health and Human Services. In essence, these guidelines represent key resources for EBP at the national level. Various professional organizations and/or groups of individuals submit the guidelines to the NGC. While the NGC has established criteria for publishing guidelines, it is still incumbent upon the reader to consider issues of quality, validity, reliability, and applicability to local situations. "Understanding the limitations of guidelines as well as their potential benefits enables clinicians to acquire a clearer view of the place of guidelines in everyday practice" (Andrews & Redmond, 2004, p. 961).

Research-Based Evidence

Sackett and colleagues (2000) defined best research evidence as clinically relevant research, based on both medical science and patient-centered clinical research. New evidence from clinical research questions previously accepted diagnostic tests and treatments, and recommends interventions that are more powerful, more accurate, more efficacious, and safer (Sackett et al.). Nursing care is more than a set of investigations and treatment interventions. Clinical nurses draw on a wide range of knowledge sources within and beyond the medical sciences, including behavioral and social sciences (Craig & Smyth, 2002). Nursing practice is informed by findings from multiple research methodologies, including interpretive phenomenology and participatory action research (Allen, Benner, Diekelmann, 1986; Benner, 1994).

A common source of evidence is the *systematic review* (Stevens, 2001). Systematic review summarizes all of the evidence related to a specific research issue using a rigorous method. It answers the question: Based on all of the available evidence, what do we know currently about this specific question (Bent, Shojania, & Saint, 2004)? *Meta-analysis* is a statistical technique that rigorously combines the findings of multiple studies on a focused question (Sackett et al., 2000). An *integrative review*, on the other hand, summarizes the findings of prior research on a particular topic and draws conclusions from the body of the literature. An *exhaustive integrative review* may meet the same standard as primary research in regard to clarity, rigor, and replication (Beyea & Nicoll, 1998). The validity of these reviews may be evaluated by asking the following questions: (a) Is the clinical question well focused? (b) Are the criteria for including articles in the review appropriate? (c) How likely is it that relevant studies were missed? (d) Are the results similar from study to study (Wolf, 2000)?

Clinical Expertise

Expert opinion is especially important in the absence of research-based studies or in instances of conflicting evidence. These may be found on professional Web sites, conference proceedings, or in peer-reviewed journals. There is also experientially based knowledge that expert clinicians possess (heuristic information) that is not available in the literature (Feuerbach & Panniers, 2003).

Patient Values and Preferences

Inclusion of the patient in decisions about his or her health care means taking into account the individual's view when interpreting and applying research evidence. It is expected that patients' willingness and ability to contribute will vary based on their health status, personal characteristics, and the nature of the decision(s) they face. The process of eliciting preferences begins by assembling an evidence-based summary of the relevant information, linking various options with outcomes, costs, benefits, and complications. Although eliciting patient preferences is a desirable goal, it may not be practical in every clinical encounter, so some selectivity is appropriate (Entwistle & O'Donnell, 2001). The inclusion of patients in appropriate areas of clinical decision-making certainly humanizes EBNP.

Other Sources of Evidence

Textbooks may provide a knowledge base, but caution is to be used based on the currency of the data and integrity of the references (Feuerbach & Panniers, 2003). Each text should be critiqued and its contents assessed by comparison with peer-reviewed journal articles and consultation with experts both from clinical practice and academe. One approach relative to the use of text references includes the use of a committee of advance practice nurses who review acceptable texts on a periodic basis.

OVERVIEW OF DISCIPLINED CLINICAL INQUIRY

Over the last two decades, tremendous advances have been made in health sciences with the development of new technology and new knowledge (Muir Gray, 2001). When a new technique is learned, even newer technology arrives, making the recently engaged learning obsolete, often before the provider has had time to assimilate previous learning (Porter-O'Grady, 2003). This health care environment demands a clear departure from traditional modes of practice inquiry (e.g., trial and error). New ways of thinking and skill sets that equip care providers with lifelong tools to enable them to systematically apply new knowledge in daily practice are needed. EBNP offers both the framework and the approach to meet these needs through DCI.

Philosophical Underpinnings and Methodology

Cognizant of both the academic and practice-based issues relative to the implementation of EBNP, the Hospitals and Clinics of the University of Texas Medical Branch (UTMB) at Galveston forged a partnership with the UTMB-

School of Nursing to develop an EBNP model using participatory action research (PAR) methodology. The model—DCI—represents the shared vision and shared experiences of nurses in clinical practice and academe (Sanares & Heliker, 2002).

PAR, based on the assumptions of critical social theory, is a collaborative research methodology designed to solve local problems that have practical and direct application to the clinical setting. These problems are addressed collaboratively among all stakeholders, those individuals most affected by the issue and its solution. Stakeholders as a group discuss the problem, identify the context, review possible solutions, choose a systematic methodology, implement the solution, and decide the criteria to be used to evaluate the process. PAR is a democratic, pragmatic, empowering, and humanizing research approach that incorporates both quantitative and qualitative methodologies of problem solving (Greenwood & Levin, 1998).

DCI is based on the philosophical assumptions of critical social theory (Friere, 1970; Habermas, 1985; Lewin, 1946). Critical social theory uses critique as a method of investigating the reality of the practices, mentalities, and institutions that make up the reality. Lewin's influence is most reflective of DCI's emphasis on the inclusion of the practitioner as the local expert in all phases of inquiry. Habermas' focus on critical knowledge based on the principles of collaboration, reflection, and communication is evident in the patterns of relationships among stakeholders. Friere's works involving an interactive learner-empowered environment influenced the design of the stakeholder-driven inquiry modules and knowledge generation and change strategies. Thus, DCI, with its principles of language (communication), locus (local environment and collaboration), leadership (change strategies), and learning becomes the pathway toward EBNP.

Context for Implementation

The fast pace at which knowledge and technology advance along with growing consumers' demands renders the content-focused traditional approach of in-house staff development programs inadequate. Valuable nursing care hours no longer can be continually short-changed by attendance at broad-based in-services and off-site seminars. No single expert or elite group of advanced practice nurses can successfully maintain the sustainability of EBNP initiatives. Neither is it realistic to expect every nurse to pursue further formal education while working full-time. The new agenda calls for a re-framing of an inquiry approach that empowers nurses to access, interpret, synthesize, and apply the most current best evidence right at the doorstep of their practice setting. DCI addresses these concerns with need-based, self-paced, and online interactive educational modules.

DCI principles are seamlessly linked with the organizational mission, nursing service philosophy, and commitment to the population it serves. To ensure feasibility and ongoing engagement at every stage of the inquiry pathway, the implementation tools and processes have built-in mechanisms that are sensitive to the workflow of the clinical nurse and the environment.

Implementation Model

Central to DCI (Figure 2.1) is the ongoing development of EBNP competencies while engaging in knowledge generation, utilization, and practice evaluation through its five cascading phases. Phase 1 provides baseline information that reflects the needs and expectations of nurses along with that of the organization. There is an emphasis on increasing awareness of one's practice and environment. Phase 2 addresses participants' interest and perceived educational needs by facilitating engagement in learning and knowledge generation strategies. Phase 3 represents the assimilation of the tools, principles, and processes acquired in Phase 2 into daily clinical decision-making and inquiry. At this point,

Figure 2.1   DCI Implementation Model

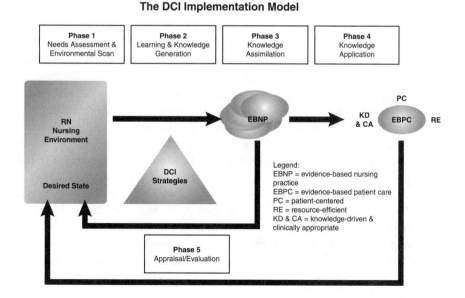

The DCI Implementation Model

a feedback loop is set in motion. If nurses demonstrate the ability to provide interventions based on the integration of the most appropriate and current best evidence, Phase 4 commences. If not, then the previous phases may be re-visited. Phase 4 is the application of evidence-based nursing interventions to specific population groups in collaboration with the other members of the care team (evidence-based patient care [EBPC]). EBP can be fully realized only if the other members of the interdisciplinary care team work in synergy within the framework of a practice based on the integration of the best evidence. Another feedback loop is set in motion at this juncture to verify the achievement of the desired outcomes. It is expected that the outcomes of care brought about by an emerging EBNP culture are expected to generate a ripple effect to other care providers as a critical mass of nurses become champions in their respective specialty arenas. Phase 5 represents ongoing critique and iterative evaluation of the process and outcomes of nursing care.

Foundational Principles

DCI has four foundational principles, the *4 Ls*, which bind the tools and processes in a seamless framework. These are: language, leadership, learning, and locus of care.

Language

Language can present a barrier to the access and understanding of research-based literature. Yet when the language of research studies is transformed into a learner-friendly format that is meaningful to the bedside nurse, the systematic inquiry inherent in EBNP is recognized as the standard for all nurses. Within the Web-based DCI program and with the use of hyperlinked text, the language of EBNP is incrementally introduced. Technical words used in the various sites are hyperlinked to a subweb called jargon that provides simple definitions, examples, and the application of concepts and principles in clinical practice. Practice standards and other relevant documentation that may clarify the topic under discussion are likewise hyperlinked. Making the "language" of EBNP nurse-friendly goes beyond familiarity with technical terms and critical documents. DCI's strategy of gradual immersion in core EBNP competencies is facilitated by exercises that provide opportunities for the immediate and practical application of concepts and principles. Tools and templates that serve as outlines and guides are included. Maintaining the continuous flow of communication and encouraging collaboration are achieved using multi-media sources. For example, a list serve may be introduced to serve as a medium to provide updates on the most current evidence-based information available online in the form of small bite news or abstracted scenarios. Allowing for various levels of technological competence, print media are also distributed to reinforce learning as well as continuing interest and engagement. DCI utilizes every available print medium in-house plus a dedicated newsletter published regularly by nurses themselves.

Leadership

The next "L" is a process of leadership that encourages mentorship and productive collegial exchanges among clinicians, educators, and researchers within and across disciplines, including the voice of the patient. Integral to DCI is the active participation of leadership at all levels and all phases. All participants can become change agents and leaders as they identify issues and participate in finding solutions that would facilitate the DCI learning journey. The visibility of administrative support is achieved by welcoming the inclusion of the chief nursing officer, directors, managers, and other leaders as either members or advisors to the DCI Core Team.

Learning

This principle refers to the nurse's personal commitment to continuous learning. Professional nurses have an equal stake in providing the highest quality, safest, and most cost-effective nursing care. Although institutions provide opportunities for continuing education units (CEUs), nurses are expected to demonstrate their professional commitment beyond the CEU obligation. DCI is a nursing inquiry model and as such creates the conditions for a teaching-learning culture.

Locus of Care

Sealing the L quadrant is the process of creating a practice culture where the locus or environment of care provides the structure, processes, and systems that support nurses' efforts to re-shape and change their practice. This evolving culture is said to have been realized when each nurse reflects on his or her day-to-day practice, using the knowledge and skills of systematic inquiry and knowledge synthesis to identify problems, find solutions to clinical issues, and strategically initiate evidence-based action plans.

When these 4 Ls are consistently in place, the attitude, knowledge, and skills of the nurse are enriched. Increased levels of interest, understanding, and commitment to the practical application of the concepts and principles of EBNP and DCI at various points of care become the normative culture. This brings about a new practice ethic whereby nurses are: (a) accessing and synthesizing the best evidence about clinical issues critical in their particular practice settings on their initiative; and (b) introducing changes and innovative practices based on the integration of the best evidence-based knowledge. In short, nurses are empowered to re-shape their practice.

Tools and Processes

DCI is an integrated practice inquiry model that supports the nurse's journey in bringing best evidence to the clinical arena. In this journey, DCI provides not only principles, but practical and actionable tools and processes required to access, critique, utilize, apply, and disseminate the most current available best evidence in one integrated framework. The model has been fine-tuned to foster pragmatic application of nursing art and science to the workflow and patterns of decision-making unique to each practice setting. This is being accomplished by jointly addressing the changing nurses' needs and patients' needs into a holistic, iterative, and proactive framework. It is holistic because learning is seamlessly integrated with knowledge generation, utilization, and application. It is iterative because continuous evaluation is built into the process. It is proactive because practice change is knowledge-driven and patient-centered. The nurse's engagement in DCI helps to create a culture of the highest level of caring vigilance. In this culture, nurses need not be prompted by occurrences or sentinel events to introduce change. Nurses become change agents, knowledge-workers, empowered, and internally motivated to re-shape their practice driven by their commitment to patient care and acquired inquiry skills. In the next section, the phases of DCI are presented from clinical practice application experiences.

PHASE 1: NEEDS ASSESSMENT, ENVIRONMENTAL SCAN, AND MOBILIZING THE STAKEHOLDERS

Nurses' Self-Needs Assessment Tool

Figure 2.2 depicts the key variables that are to be considered in determining the current and desired needs of nurses in the organization. Using a structured survey format, nurses are cued to reflect on the context of their practice (professional, institutional, societal) and helped to become more astute regarding their current experience, knowledge, learning needs, and areas of interest related to research and EBNP. Each of these key items (knowledge, experience, attitude, learning needs) have several indicators that are evaluated using a 5-point Likert-

Figure 2.2 Key Variables of Self-Needs Assessment

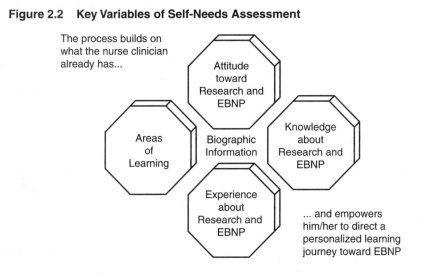

The process builds on what the nurse clinician already has...

Attitude toward Research and EBNP

Knowledge about Research and EBNP

Areas of Learning

Biographic Information

Experience about Research and EBNP

... and empowers him/her to direct a personalized learning journey toward EBNP

type scale and open ended questions. The survey was developed with input from clinicians and nurse managers.

Environmental Scan

Along with the needs survey, Phase 1 calls for a scan of nursing workflow patterns, institutional core values and mission, and the requirements of the current health care arena. The individual and environmental components of the assessment are then analyzed to identify strengths, weaknesses, opportunities, and threats that may affect the entire practice arena. Processes are identified that may facilitate or disrupt the creation of an ethic of care and a culture (locus or environment of care) that provides the structure, processes, and systems supportive of nurses' efforts to re-shape their practice.

Cultures do not turn sharply with the pages of the calendar; they evolve. By becoming aware of what is changing today, we know what we must improve upon tomorrow (Bennis, 2000). Nurses, therefore, must monitor and critique advances in biomedical science, new clinical care technologies, and changes in population sociodemographics and their impact on nursing practice. Nursing's Agenda for the Future (2002) recognized that uniting nursing organizations to advance EBP would move the profession forward in quantum leaps. Nurses must be aware of the significance of the 2003 Institute of Medicine (IOM) report, authored by a multidisciplinary group of health professionals across the nation, that identified the five *core competencies* of all health professionals, one of which is to employ EBP. (The other four are: provide patient-centered care, work in an interdisciplinary team, apply quality improvement, and utilize informatics.) These external forces are to be interpreted within concurrent streams of change occurring in health care at the regional and community levels. As the professional and environmental awareness of the nurse is heightened, these resources and directives become imperative and significant.

These external forces are carefully reviewed vis-à-vis the internal dynamics of nursing workflow, patterns of clinical decision-making, professional relationships, and other support systems in care delivery. The vision and program priorities of those in top leadership positions are compared with that of the nursing enterprise and finally to unit-specific priorities, all of which are woven with the common concern of quality care. A mere statement that EBNP is a key strategic initiative to achieve excellence is not enough. True commitment is manifested in the flow and allocation of resources. Dedicated time for the core team and participating nurses is exceedingly important. Access to major databases (i.e., Cochrane, CINAHL, and Medline) and other internet sources (National Guidelines Clearing House, TRIP, and Joanna Briggs Foundation) is indispensable. If these are not currently available in nursing service, special efforts are needed to include these tools in the organizational budget cycle.

Data Management

The self-needs report assessment and environmental scan data are analyzed in parallel to generate the most accurate and complementary information and provide the knowledge base needed to proceed to Phase 2. Current strengths and needs are systematically compared with the current and desired nursing practice environments. Data are reported to all stakeholders in user-friendly language and questions are answered. The current state is described and plotted alongside the desired state. If gaps exist, the new vision and viable strategies needed to achieve the desired state as defined by the nurses ensure a successful initiative with innovative nursing interventions. Thus, the voices of the nurses are indeed being heard and valued.

At the individual level, the nurse uses the results as a guide in customizing one's professional journey toward EBNP. At the unit and organizationwide level, the results are used in designing an EBNP program. Nursing leaders guide the development of clinical nurses and promote professional advancement. This accountability is aligned with the organizational mission and program priorities. Therefore, it is critically important to systematically map out the cost and value of the EBNP initiative with the data-driven parameters collected in the self-needs assessment and environmental scan.

Knowledge and Skill Set Gaps

A gap between knowledge and skill sets is likely to exist if the organization has a greater percentage of nurses whose basic nursing education has not systematically integrated the principles and utilization of EBNP. A number of nursing educational programs have begun introducing EBNP strategies in their undergraduate nursing curricula. EBP literature and continuing education opportunities have also increased exponentially over the last decade. However, several studies continue to reiterate barriers that hinder nurses from ascribing to EBP (Beyea & Nicoll, 1997; Funk, Tornquist, & Champagne, 1995; McCleary & Brown, 2003; Newman, Papadopoulos, & Sigsworth, 1998; Retsas, 2000; Rutledge, Ropka, Greene, Nail, & Mooney, 1998). Some of the most notable are inaccessibility of the language of research, insufficient employer support, and inadequate knowledge about EBP. Interestingly, the 2003 IOM report noted that the "support systems that will help access and utilize the new knowledge and technology in an accessible format at the point of care are currently not widely available" (p. 33).

Mobilizing the Stakeholders

Successful adoption of DCI as a framework for EBNP requires a shift in thinking. New relationship patterns among all stakeholders must develop. Nurses in leadership positions and nurses at the bedside collaborate as they consciously create a new shared vision of the role of nursing in the organization. This is complemented by a firm resolve to engage in shared experiences as the vision becomes realized in the practice setting. If nursing service is operating under the umbrella of an academic medical center, collegial partnerships with nursing faculty in academe are established during this stage. Interconnectedness and open communication among all stakeholders ensure common ownership and accountability during the development, implementation, and evaluation phases. Respectful recognition of individual areas of expertise and concerns and the interdependence of professional roles acknowledges: (1) nursing leaders as facilitators of resources; (2) nursing faculty as mentors; and (3) frontline staff as experts of "local" clinical knowledge and co-creators of new knowledge.

The new patterns of relationships (Figure 2.3) depart from traditional hierarchal organizations as the stakeholders begin relating in a circular motion and interconnectedness as desired outcomes are defined and evaluated. Stakeholders

Figure 2.3   Relationship Patterns of Stakeholders

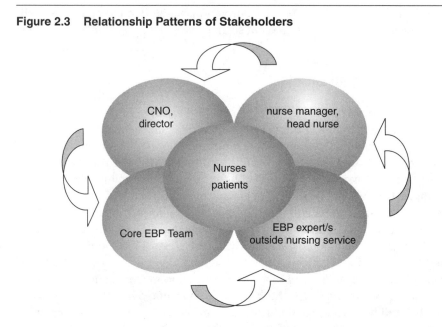

are engaged at the very outset consistent with the DCI principle: EBNP is jointly shaped by those who create it, use it, and evaluate it.

The Core DCI/EBNP Team

This team is the prime mover of the initiative and may be organized in a variety of ways depending upon the organization. Participation is open to all nurses. Team members who exemplify professional commitment and motivation are sought to introduce and model the process of DCI in the practice setting. A clinical nurse with practical knowledge of issues in each arena champions the inquiry effort. Each core member is a respected and trusted colleague within the nursing enterprise by virtue of demonstrated knowledge, attitude, and skills, and not by virtue of de facto authority alone. It is desirable that the leader of the core team be masters-prepared and have experience in research, EBP, or project management. In the absence of these credentials, the identified leader can be successful with ongoing mentorship, successful completion of the DCI Web-based learning modules, or attendance at EBP conferences or course offerings.

A core team leader, appointed as the EBNP Program Manager, may operate within a mandated organizational matrix structure that allows all members of the team to contribute and participate in the DCI process. This structure offers flexibility and greater latitude in engaging the clinical experts from various nursing specialties. The Core DCI/EBNP team may initially be organized as a special task force with a mandate and support from administrative leadership. Members of the core team should represent the various stakeholders.

Nurses

Nurses are the frontline staff providing complex nursing interventions and making hundreds of clinical decisions every day (Swan & Boruch, 2004). While the partnership among the key stakeholders is aimed at equality of ownership and accountability, the nature of the nursing role places these frontline care providers in a strategic position. It is within these daily face-to-face encounters with patients, their families and significant others, and the institutional system that problems are identified and solved. The intensity and demands inherent in this role require all ways of knowing, including experience, esthetics, personal knowing, patient perspective, ethical knowing, socioeconomic knowing, and clinical reasoning as well as the ability to access and appropriately utilize the most current and valid knowledge and technology at the point of care (Higgs, Burn, & Jones, 2001). That is why nurses share center stage with the patients who are the ultimate beneficiary of the EBNP initiative.

Pool of Experts

These advisors and collaborators are invited as mentors and coaches throughout the DCI journey. The knowledge and skill to critique research-based evidence may require external experts for guidance and tutoring. Experts may be identified from another sector of the organization, affiliated academic units, or outsourced through joint-venture agreements until internal expertise is fully developed.

Nursing Leadership

The leaders are composed of (a) the Chief Nursing Officer or Directors, who provide the strategic and long-term vision and resources; and (b) first-line managers and /or head nurses, who provide unit level and short-term goals and resources. Time is one of the critical resources that can either facilitate or undermine an EBNP initiative like the DCI model. It is therefore imperative to obtain a mandate from leadership at the outset. Informal leaders are likewise identified and welcomed. There may always be detractors or skeptics; planning for this contingency lessens unpredictable challenges. Leadership buy-in is best secured when outcomes are demonstrated. This is accomplished by starting small, that is, pilot testing in one or two nursing units where the core team has clinical expertise. The pilot unit serves as a demonstration area that establishes the visible impact of a nursing inquiry model and the viability of EBNP. The pilot also demonstrates the credibility of the core team and the feasibility of the structure and process prior to large-scale implementation.

Other Members of the Care Team

Bringing the above-mentioned stakeholders to a "level table" at the very beginning is key to the smooth introduction and sustainability of the DCI/EBNP initiative. At this point, the stakeholders mentioned have been primarily nurses. Yet patient care is multidisciplinary and outcomes are best achieved through collaboration. Ideally, EBP initiatives should occur concurrently in the other disciplines—especially among physicians—to achieve a maximum impact. DCI as an inquiry model crosses all disciplines and has been shown to be highly effective especially within the inquiry tracks of research studies, journal clubs, and seminars. Nurses are encouraged to actively seek partnerships with the other disciplines as co-investigators in primary research, resource persons in journal clubs, participants in clinical inquiry sessions, or as consultants/validation experts in the development of practice standards.

Ongoing connecting conversations among these groups and individuals enhance the success of the DCI initiative.

PHASE 2: LEARNING AND KNOWLEDGE GENERATION

The results of Phase 1 serve as the basis to develop the structure, processes, and systems to actualize EBNP in the practice setting. Attention to the results of Phase 1 ensures that the DCI/EBNP initiative is tailored fit to meet the needs and requirements of the patients, staff, and organization.

The Learning Modules

Within the DCI framework, nurses demonstrate a willingness to match organizational support by making a personal commitment to continuous learning and assuming the role of inquiry-based problem solvers. Nurses already in the work force may effectively challenge conventional wisdom and become co-creators of new knowledge. To meet the specific learning needs of individual nurses, DCI offers on-line, need-based, self-paced EBNP educational modules. These modules must always be responsive to the changing needs of the nurse. Hence, revisions are ongoing.

DCI's strategy of gradual immersion into clinical inquiry and EBNP competency is facilitated by interactive exercises that provide opportunities for the immediate application of concepts and principles while serving as a working template for a predetermined EBNP product/outcome. A number of tools and templates that serve as outlines and guides are included. Each Web site page provides easy access to a Web master who can respond to questions or facilitate referral to appropriate experts as applicable.

Each of the modules has a specific focus of learning inquiry as outlined in Table 2.1. These learning activities may be completed independently. Several modules offer Type I continuing nursing education credit.

Table 2.1   DCI Learning Inquiry Modules

Title	Focus of Inquiry
Becoming a reflective nurse clinician	Value, process, & attributes of reflective nursing practice
Identifying clinical issues & establishing priorities	Process & principles of identifying & prioritizing clinical issues sensitive to nursing interventions
Identifying practice standards & establishing priorities	Processes, principles & tools in identifying priority practice standards
Translating clinical issues into a researchable problem/focused question	Process & principles of developing & refining clinical issues into a testable problem statements/questions
Accessing the best evidence	Process of identifying & locating sources of best evidence
Evaluating research studies	Process & principles of reading & critiquing research studies
Utilizing the best evidence	Process & tools for appraising EBNP standards; principles & processes of resolving conflicting evidence; & integrating best evidence
Strategic thinking & action planning	Value, principles, & process of strategic thinking & action planning

Multiple Modalities

Learning is an individualized process. While some individuals prefer a structured small group teaching/learning approach, others prefer a self-paced solitary format. There are learners who thrive with Web-based instruction and others who maintain that traditional face-to-face or written materials serve them well. It is for this reason that a multi-media approach is used throughout this initiative. The availability and best combination of high touch and low touch approaches, as shown in Figure 2.4, is offered. The environmental scan provides cues identifying which combination works well in particular health settings. Organizations that are unable to access the DCI Web site can design learning pathways customized to their needs by using printed materials.

Learning-Knowledge Generation Pathways

The pathways offer participants ways of generating knowledge and increasing their skill levels using the information gained through module activity. Nurses have the option of becoming involved with any of the pathways, or combination of pathways, based on their personal interest and capability (Table 2.2). To increase understanding, they may use the reflective questions (Table 2.3). There are varying degrees of involvement in these pathways, ranging from assuming a leadership role to becoming a member of the team.

Figure 2.4   DCI Multimedia Support Interface

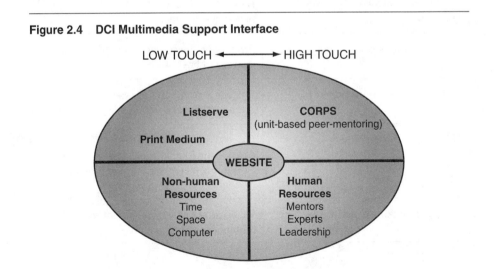

Table 2.2   DCI/EBNP Pathways

Pathway	Focus of Inquiry	Method of Inquiry
Developing evidence-based practice standards	Clinical practice issues with valued clinical & institutional significance	Accessing, integrating, & utilizing the most current sources of best evidence in the development/update of practice standards
Conducting research studies	Practice issues with valued clinical & institutional significance	Research process or integrative reviews of the literature focused on a specific research problem
Preparing notes for nurses	Clinical practice issues with valued clinical & institutional significance	Accessing, integrating, & utilizing the most current sources of best evidence in preparing a concise evidence-based fact sheet for nurses
Forming journal clubs	Published research studies on clinical issues of high volume, high intensity, & high risk	Review & critique of pre-selected research studies & determination of its applicability to the practice setting
Organizing clinical inquiry sessions	This is a dialogue involving reflection on actual care provided. Focus is on rationale & outcome of current practices.	Reflections on care, identifying both the problems encountered & the successes achieved along the care continuum. Evidence-based data such as expert opinion & research are used during this forum.
Becoming a peer-mentor	Leadership potential of a cohort of RNs to serve as unit-based DCI peer-mentors to facilitate nurses' competency in DCI	Leading, mentoring, & tracking peers' DCI journey

Table 2.3   Reflections on Pathway Choices

Strategic Questions	Pathway Choice
Am I someone who would read and critique the scholarly works of others and brainstorm with my peers regarding their applicability to my practice setting?	Journal club
Am I someone who would scientifically investigate causes, relationships, and solutions of priority clinical issues?	Research study
Am I someone who would organize my peers, seek expert opinion, and engage my colleagues in a structured discussion of actual nursing care provided?	Clinical inquiry session
Am I someone who would integrate the best evidence in a one-page concise format that is understandable to my peers?	Notes for nurses
Am I someone who would enjoy facilitating the development of the evidence-based competency levels of my peers?	Peer-mentorship
Am I someone who would like to review/update/develop standards of care that are based on the integration of the best evidence?	Evidence-based practice standards

As the nurse advances in EBNP competencies, he or she can volunteer to be a peer-mentor.

Each of the above pathways is discussed below.

Research

Research is one of the pathways that nurses can choose depending on individual interest level. Engaging in the research pathway will help acquire understanding and beginning skills to use the research methodology, identify resources, and establish partnerships that set the tone for an inquiry-based practice. It focuses on the acquisition of foundational knowledge and skills in preparing a research proposal. The study can be in the form of clinical research or an integrative review focused upon a clinical issue with valued clinical and institutional significance. It is learner-directed and nurses are personally responsible for tracking their level of research competency and in determining how much coaching is needed to achieve goals. This is determined by the result of individual "self assessment." The pathway incorporates a mentoring approach as nurses are immersed in the acquisition and application of the key elements of the research process.

Journal Clubs

A journal club is review and critique of research-based studies related to specific clinical issues. At the end of this pathway, the nurse is expected to facilitate the review and critique of a research study and evaluate its implications and application in practice. If the group decides that the findings of the study may be considered for a change in practice, the nurse leading the journal club session is expected to prepare an action plan. The action plan may include finding additional evidence-based information that supports or negates the findings. At the end of the session, the facilitator, in collaboration with the unit-based journal club coordinator, will prepare a brief summary using the journal club template link and share conclusions with those unable to attend the journal club.

Clinical Inquiry Sessions

This pathway allows nurses to reflect on actual care provided for a particular patient. The problems encountered and the successes achieved along the care continuum are identified. Evidence-based data are referenced as nurses engage in the inquiry process, exploring the causes and solutions sensitive to nursing interventions. At the end of the session, nurses are expected to acquire better understandings and practice perspectives. Insights gained in the session lead nurses toward the exploration of opportunities for EBNP. The inquiry session is designed to serve as a reflective lens for practitioners in forms including: (a) patient case presentation; (b) multidiscipline case review and analysis; and (c) multidiscipline patient care planning.

Notes for Nurses

Notes for nurses focuses on practices that address the questions, "why are we doing what we're doing?" Nurses engaged in this pathway utilize the DCI process in summarizing best evidence derived from the integration of research, expert opinion, pathophysiologic rationale, patient perspectives, and other recognized sources of nursing knowledge. Its primary purpose is to share with peers the most current, valid, and reliable evidence-based knowledge about nursing practices. New knowledge is presented in a concise one-page summary that nurse clinicians can quickly peruse amidst a high intensity care environment.

Peer-Mentorship

This pathway prepares nurses to become part of a cohort serving as unit-based DCI/EBNP champions. A peer-mentor coaches colleagues as they learn the principles, processes, and tools of the DCI inquiry model through Web-based learning. The DCI mentoring tree is introduced as the mentee develops optimum skill levels and an EBNP knowledge base. The nurse peer-mentor is a recognized practitioner in her specialty and is not only concerned with personal and professional development, but equally with the growth and development of his or her peers. After agreeing to become a peer-mentor, a meeting is called to discuss Web-based mentoring.

Evidence-Based Practice Standards

Unlike physicians, nurses are not as free to change their practice without the support of the organization. If EBNP is to become integral in the health care culture, an organized effort to understand organizational influences and to develop an infrastructure that promotes EBP is critical (Foxcroft & Cole, 2004). The principles, processes, and tools of DCI are sensitive to any existing organizational climate. If the shared vision and experiences of all stakeholders are directly linked with essential nursing functions, the initiative sustains itself. Essential nursing functions in this context refer to nursing activities that have been traditionally accepted by both clinicians and management as a component of nursing practice. The most notable of these essential functions are the development of practice standards, provision of patient teaching, and quality improvement projects.

Despite significant strides accorded to clinical practice guideline development at the national level, there is a dearth of systematic studies that apply EBP/EBNP in the appraisal and development of practice standards at the organizational level. As a predetermined level of safe nursing practice, nursing services have invested significant time, talent, and resources to develop and update standards of care. Ensuring that nursing practice standards keep pace with the most current best evidence remains a continuing challenge. If the authoritative statements guiding day-to-day nursing practice are not keeping pace with the most current best evidence, potential adverse effects on patient care exist.

The evidence-based practice standards (EBPS) pathway may be completed in 24 to 32 hours over a four-month period (Table 2.4). The formalized structure and processes facilitate the: (a) integration of EBNP competencies in the

Table 2.4 Exemplar of an Evidence-Based Practice Standards (EBPS) Pathway

Pathway	Areas of Learning	Outcomes
Introduction	Instituting evidence-based practice standards system	Expressed understanding
Stages	Stage of achieving an EBPS management system	Expressed understanding
Game Plan	The game plan	Expressed understanding
Pathway 1: Establishing baseline competency	Conducting needs self-assessment	Expressed understanding & completed reflective questions
Pathway 2: Acquiring basic knowledge	Evaluating EBNP (a) why EBNP (b) impact to the organization (c) what is DCI? (d) getting familiar with EBP/EBNP jargon (e) reflective questions	Expressed understanding & completed reflective questions
Pathway 3: Acquiring basic knowledge & skills	Instituting evidence-based practice standards Module #1: Identifying PS & determining priorities Module #2: Translating a clinical issue into a focused question Module #3: Accessing the evidence-based knowledge Module #4: Evaluating research articles Module #5: Utilizing the best evidence	Completed exercises & completed reflective questions Appraised/developed EBPS
Pathway 4: Acquiring basic skills	Disseminating EBPS	Designed/Conducted Dissemination Strategies
Pathway 5: Acquiring basic skills	Evaluating impact	Completed Impact Evaluation

Advancement and Performance Standards and Evaluation criteria appropriate for each level of nursing practice; and (b) incorporation of DCI/EBNP structure and processes in the development and update of standards of care (Figure 2.5).

The resources needed to individually and collectively engage nurses in continuous learning are identified and used judiciously. Web-based learning is used and is complemented by both virtual and live coaching from clinical and academic experts. At the point at which nurses completed the EBPS, the process of knowledge assimilation in nursing practice (Phase 3 of the DCI model) begins.

PHASE 3: KNOWLEDGE ASSIMILATION IN EVIDENCE-BASED NURSING PRACTICE

Knowledge assimilation is the process whereby EBNP becomes integrated within individual practice patterns and the practice systems of nursing service. In Phase 1, individual nurses become self-reflective regarding their abilities and learning needs that serve as their personal guide toward Phase 2. Concurrently,

---

Figure 2.5   Evidence-Based Practice Standards System

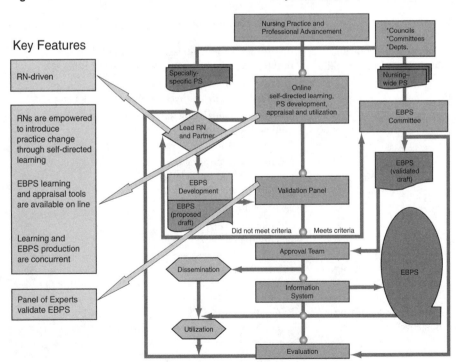

the DCI Core Team conducts an environmental scan to identify organizational characteristics, processes, and infrastructures. The learning modules and pathways in Phase 2 offer need-based, self-directed, stepwise processes of acquiring EBNP competencies along with the immediate application of these skills. If these abilities and their applications become integral to daily nursing practice, knowledge assimilation is said to have been realized. It is, however, important to note that the rate and level of knowledge assimilation is not only a function of individual nurses' abilities and motivation, but equally a function of the organizational system in which nurses practice.

Individual Practice Patterns

After completing a chosen DCI pathway, a nurse is expected to critically reflect on his or her practice and apply the acquired EBNP skill set in daily clinical decision-making. This means the nurse is becoming both a reflective and outcomes-oriented practitioner. The nurse routinely monitors experiences and develops increasing levels of self knowledge, striving toward greater understanding of the commitment to achieve desirable work in everyday practice (Johns & Freshwater, 1998). The nurse becomes open to new possibilities of nursing practice, and routinely engages in the systematic examination and understanding of how the most current best evidence can inform a particular area of practice. These patterns of practice lead to the achievement of EBNP. DCI acknowledges that EBNP may be demonstrated in varying degrees based on the level of a nurse's clinical practice. For example, in organizations with a clinical ladder, expert level nurses are expected to have a higher degree of knowledge and skill in synthesizing and applying the best evidence in particular patient care situations compared to a novice nurse. "Nurses apply the newly acquired practice patterns in making clinical decisions relative to: (a) intervention effectiveness (e.g., choosing among multiple interventions, which patient will most benefit from the intervention, and the best time to employ particular interventions); (b) communication (e.g., choices relating to ways of delivering and receiving information to and from patients, families & colleagues); (c) service organization, delivery, and management (e.g., decisions concerning the configuration or processes of service delivery); (d) experience, understanding, and hermeneutics (e.g., relates to the interpretation of cues in the process of care) (Thompson, Cullum, McCaughan, Sheldon, & Raynor, 2000, p. 69)."

Practice Systems of Nursing Service

Little systematic attention has been devoted to the elements required to operationalize EBP in the nursing literature beyond creation of a limited number of research-based practices or procedures. In particular, little attention has been paid to the elements required to integrate EBNP into the daily lives and routines of professional nurses (Stetler, 2003, p. 97). The characteristics of the "locus of care" greatly influence the sustainability of newly acquired practice patterns.

If the benefits of EBNP are to become widespread in health services, organized efforts to promote EBNP are crucial (Foxcroft & Cole, 2004). It is for this reason that DCI advocates the link between EBNP initiatives and essential nursing functions. This strategy facilitates the creation of an infrastructure for EBNP. By the same token, new knowledge does not have any value unless it reaches the intended users. DCI provides strategies for transforming new knowledge into an accessible format that nurses can utilize at the point of care. It is not reasonable to expect all nurses in every situation to access, critique, and integrate best evidence. DCI offers organized efforts and a medium where sources of best evidence are shared and disseminated.

PHASE 4: KNOWLEDGE APPLICATION IN EVIDENCE-BASED PATIENT CARE

Applying the Best Evidence to Patient Care

EBNP and EBPC may be argued to occur simultaneously in real time. However, within the DCI framework, EBNP and EBPC become two outcomes on a continuum, whereby EBPC is evaluated by the quality of care already received by the patient. Patient care is interdisciplinary and multidisciplinary. Within this perspective, EBPC is defined as the optimum interface of clinically appropriate, resource-efficient, and patient-centered care. A nurse who has acquired EBNP competencies is expected to identify and provide a unique contribution as a collegial member of the health care team. This unique contribution defines the nature of the patient issue that lies within the domain of nursing practice. While it is recognized that overlaps of functions exist, nursing, like medicine, has specific domains of practice that are reflective of the profession. For example, when deciding which antibiotic would be most effective for a particular disease, a physician may utilize the Cochrane's hierarchy of evidence (Table 2.5). In this case, a well-conducted systematic review of randomized controlled trials (RCTs) offers the best evidence. For the patient receiving the prescribed medication, the nurse might go beyond the Cochrane hierarchy to make a series of clinical decisions based on a number of the issues.

Table 2.6 shows the nature of the decisions the nurse has to make and the gold standards he or she is going to use. The example above is not intended to be ex-

Table 2.5   Cochrane Collaboration's Levels of Evidence

Level I: Systematic review of well-designed randomized controlled trials (RCT)
Level II: RCT
Level III: Nonrandomized clinical trials
Level IV: Well designed nonexperimental studies
Level V: Opinions of respected authorities based upon clinical evidence, reports of expert committees
Level VI: Someone's opinion

Table 2.6   Nursing Decisions

Clinical Issues	Gold standard
Allergy	Patient's voice
Drug interaction	RCT
IV flush solution	Well-conducted nonrandomized studies
Site selection	Clinical expertise
Anxiety over a needlestick	Patient
Noncompliance with treatment	Well-conducted qualitative study

haustive, but only an illustration that a prescribed method of hierarchy/grading system is not adequate to address the real world of nursing practice. Not only because there are few good RCTs that can support nursing interventions, but a substantial number of patient issues sensitive to nursing interventions cannot be appropriately nor adequately validated through RCT. As one nursing EBP scholar, states,

> The practice context is complex, people are complex, and clinicians are complex. The best evidence will most probably come in different forms, in different situations,

and context...Knowing how to decipher this complexity...and knowing how to match situation and context with appropriate evidence, will perhaps be the most important requirement of the 21st-century practicing nurse (Estabrooks, 1998, p. 30).

This wisdom tells us that nursing is not prescriptive. The essential components of nursing knowledge—its art and science—are integrated, interdependent, and complementary. They inform and enhance each other, and cannot be easily extrapolated or separated (Bailey, 2004). Nursing practice draws from various sources of knowledge and multiple ways of knowing.

To provide EBPC, nurses need a full understanding of the complexity and the uniqueness of each patient care encounter. Nurses can provide such care using disciplined inquiry and continuous reflection on the principles, processes, and tools of DCI.

PHASE 5: IMPACT EVALUATION

The pilot implementations of DCI indicated that unit-based peer-mentors facilitate the achievement of EBNP. However, the ability of the peer-mentor to impact a critical mass of nurses is difficult to achieve unless a supportive organizational infrastructure is also established. According to Rogers' (1995, p. 313) definition of critical mass, as the "point at which enough individuals have adopted an innovation that the innovation's further rate of adoption becomes self-sustaining," the impact of DCI is evaluated at both the unit and organizational levels. There will be units that adopt DCI at a faster rate than others. Understanding this phenomenon is important in the study of factors that serve as a model for the lagging units. This approach is especially important in large academic centers, where there is a high degree of specialization and spatial factors that decrease nurses' socialization processes across various specialties.

An Iterative Process

An iterative evaluation process is integral to the DCI process. Empowerment evaluation is utilized to determine nurses' satisfaction with the DCI journey. It has been argued that "in order to ensure that programs have a lasting effect, they need to be conceptualized, negotiated, run, and evaluated jointly by all stakeholders" (Van Vlaenderen & Nkwinti, as cited in Van Vlaenderen, 2001, p. 343). As such, empowerment evaluation will be utilized alongside other objective measures. Nurses are periodically asked to conduct self-evaluations and reflect critically on practice issues as well as the process of finding solutions and taking corrective actions.

Empowerment Evaluation

Empowerment evaluation is the use of evaluative concepts, techniques, and findings to foster improvement. It employs both qualitative and quantitative methodologies and is attentive to empowering processes and outcomes. The process is empowering if it helps individuals develop skills to become problem solvers and decision-makers. Empowerment outcomes refer to consequences of participants' attempts to gain greater control of their practice or the effects of interventions designed to empower the participants. It is designed to help people help themselves and improve their programs using a form of self-evaluation and reflection (Fetterman, Kaftarian, & Wandersman, 1996). Consistent with these principles, DCI offers self-evaluation tools that provide nurses with the ability to track their achievements and areas for improvement. The following paragraphs describe some of these tools that may be used for evaluation purposes.

Tool #1: Evaluating the Culture

Nurses reflect on the factors that facilitate or hamper the evolution of an EBNP culture based on their personal experience during the DCI journey using a five-point Likert-type scale. Objectively, the evolving culture is expected to have been realized in the practice arena when nurses start routinely reflecting on their day-to-day practice using systematic inquiry to identify problems, create solutions, and strategically initiate evidence-based action plans.

Tool #2: Evaluating Competency

The second area of empowerment evaluation focuses on nurses' competencies in acquiring EBNP abilities through Web-based self-directed learning. The expected competencies correspond to the various sections of the learning journey: identifying clinical issues and determining priorities; translating clinical issues into a researchable problem/focused question; accessing the evaluating research studies; using the evidence-based knowledge; resolving conflicting evidence; synthesizing the evidence; disseminating new knowledge; and evaluating impact. A Likert scale with four levels of competencies (awareness, beginning skills, independence, and mentorship) is used.

Tool #3: Evaluating Productivity

Nurses' productivity is reported in terms of the nature and degree of their participation and capacity to develop strategies that facilitate the dissemination and application of best evidence in a specialty area. Nurses report in which capacity they participated: as a member, resource person, team leader, or mentor.

Tool #4: Evaluating Satisfaction

This involves appraising the degree to which the learning journey met one's personal needs and explores the satisfaction levels of patients impacted by the initiative. Specific clinical impact is assessed using outcomes or population-based research methods. Self-appraisal of personal levels of satisfaction is reported by evaluation of the newly acquired practice ethic in increasing one's capability to provide evidence-based nursing interventions. Personal satisfaction includes: reflection on competency to systematically impact practice; being in a workplace that promotes a culture of excellence; becoming a collegial partner in caring; and other benefits gained as a result of an ongoing learning journey.

Objective Tools

Self-evaluation and reflection are complemented by objective evaluation tools. These include electronic monitoring of self-directed learning, review of on-going patient satisfaction surveys, and other reports. Patient and family perspectives of self-efficacy related to understanding illness and promoting healthy lifestyles will in turn be indicative of their adherence to teaching and learning strategies based on evidence-based knowledge.

REFLECTIONS ON THE PILOT PROJECTS

The series of pilot projects that gave birth to the DCI model demonstrated a gap in knowledge and skill sets relative to EBNP. It is for this reason that knowledge generation may not immediately become evident. The advance practice nurses can acquire or may already possess EBNP competencies. However, the goal of the DCI model is to engage not simply a few, but a critical mass of front-line nurses at various levels of competency in knowledge generation, utilization, and application. There may be nurses who are not yet up to the challenge, but this is a decision for each individual nurse. The needs assessment is the evidence-based tool for this decision-making. If the decision is to move forward, a learning opportunity is made available on a "one-stop" Web site that is easily accessed at a place and time convenient for the individual. This approach challenged nurses to explore their possibilities while making themselves professionally accountable.

Integrating EBP into Nursing Structures and Systems

Integrating learning into the everyday work flow processes of professional practice is challenging but not impossible. The initial years of implementation demonstrated a slow progression of learning. Internal motivations as well as baseline education were recognized as determinants. A more actionable aspect of this issue was the re-tooling of the processes that enabled nurses' ongoing engagement. One action agenda was to develop unit-based peer-mentors with whom nurses could regularly dialogue at work. This approach was tested in two specialty units. The intensity of the method and the amount of time required to achieve the outcomes in a short period became problematic. Building EBNP expertise at the mentor level requires intense coaching and dedicated time; however, the complexity of the nursing work flow would not permit time to achieve this expertise. With the increasing active involvement of the chief nursing executive, the success, challenges, and opportunities of the DCI projects were revisited. Consequently, the pragmatic approach was to: (1) systematically link the EBNP initiatives with essential nursing service functions; and (2) integrate EBNP abilities into the Clinical Advancement Program Performance Standards and Evaluation Criteria appropriate for each nurse clinician. These two-prong approaches not only increased the probability of positive acceptance and successful introduction of EBNP changes, but ensured sustainability of DCI over time. The required nursing service functions identified included the development of EBPSs, the provision of evidence-based patient teaching notes, and the creation of quality improvement initiatives.

SUMMARY

People who change not merely the content of a particular discipline but its practice and focus are not only innovators, but leaders (Bennis, 2000, p. 33). DCI has indeed produced leaders. From its modest beginnings as a single specialty-based project, frontline nurses engaged in DCI have since published their personal experiences in DCI-sponsored research studies, journal clubs, and evidence-based notes for nurses in the academic medical center's quarterly nursing publication. Two teams of bedside nurses received local Sigma Theta Tau International chapter grant awards for their research projects. Examples of nurse-driven research using the DCI model are: (1) a quasiexperimental study on music as a nonpharmacologic intervention in decreasing the anxiety levels of patients during conscious sedation surgery; (2) a comparative study on the effectiveness of three temperature devices; and (3) a descriptive study on the factors affecting early postoperative mobility among adult patients. EBNP poster presentations were also developed addressing the following projects: (a) prevention of deep vein thrombosis during surgery; (b) utilization of brushless operating room scrub; and (c) nonpharmacologic intervention to allay anxiety during conscious sedation surgery. Examples of clinical issues addressed in the development of EBNP standards are: guidelines for a nurse-led clinic; infection control; patency and risk factors relative to intravenous and arterial lines; prevention of deep vein thrombosis during the intra-operative period; determination of nasogastric tube placement; tracheostomy management; and efficacy of antibiotic wash during surgery. DCI as an EBNP model has been presented at national conferences and published in a peer-reviewed journal. It is significant that immersion in DCI assisted nurses' advancement on the hospital's clinical ladder. These nurses are evolving as unit-based champions and peer-mentors not because of external forces, but because they became committed to and valued EBNP.

DCI started small. Over time, as increasing numbers of nurses participated and with leadership's active engagement and support, DCI has now evolved as a practice strategy in achieving nursing excellence across our nursing enterprise. Some of the system's revisions include: (1) integration of EBNP abilities into the Clinical Advancement Program and Performance Standards and Evaluation criteria appropriate for each level of nursing practice; (2) adoption of a transition structure and process for updating and developing nursing standards of care; and (3) creation of Office of Nursing Practice and Professional Advancement with a Program Manager for EBNP as a guide for educational offerings and system's development.

ACKNOWLEDGMENTS

The authors would like to acknowledge the support, encouragement, and advice of two leaders from the University of Texas Medical Branch at Galveston—Hospitals and Clinics.

David Marshall, RN, MSN, JD, CNAA
Executive Director and Chief Nursing Officer

Phyllis Waters, PhD, RN, MS
Nursing Director
Nursing Practice and Professional Advancement

REFERENCES

Allen, D., Benner, P., & Diekelmann, N. (1986). Three paradigms for nursing research: Methodological implications. In P. Chinn (Ed), *Nursing Research Methodology: Issues and Implementations* (pp. 23–38). Rockville, MD: Aspen.

Andrews, E. J., & Redmond, H. P. (2004). A review of clinical guidelines. *British Journal of Surgery, 91,* 956–964.

Bailey, S. (2004). Nursing knowledge in integrated care. *Nursing Standard, 18*(44), 38–41.

Benner, P. (Ed.) (1994). *Interpretive Phenomenology: Embodiment, Caring, and Ethics in Health Care and Illness.* Thousand Oaks, CA: Sage.

Benner, P. (1999). Nursing leadership for the millennium: Claiming the wisdom & worth of clinical practice. *Nursing and Health Care Perspectives, 20*(6), 312–319.

Benner, P. (2000). The wisdom of caring practice. *Nursing Management, 6*(10), 32–37.

Bennis, W. (2000). *Managing the Dream: Reflections on Leadership and Change.* Cambridge, MA: Perseus Publishing.

Bent, S., Shojania, K., & Saint, S. (2004). The use of systematic reviews and meta-analysis in infection control and hospital epidemiology. *American Journal of Infection Control, 32,* 246–254.

Berg, A. O. (2000). Dimension of evidence. In J. P. Geyman, R. A. Deyo, & S. D. Ramsey (Eds), *Evidence-Based Clinical Practice: Concepts and Approaches.* Boston: Butterworth-Heinemann.

Beyea, S. C., & Nicoll, L. H. (1997). Barriers to and facilitators of research utilization in perioperative nursing practice. *AORN Journal, 65,* 830–831.

Beyea, S. C., & Nicoll, L. H. (1998). Writing an integrative review. *AORN Journal, 67,* 877–880.

Carper, B. (1978). Fundamental patterns of knowing in nursing. *Advances in Nursing Science, 1,* 13–23.

Craig, J. V., & Smyth, R. (Eds.) (2002). *The Evidence-Based Practice Manual for Nurses.* London: Churchill Livingstone.

Drucker, P. F. (2002). *Managing in the Next Society.* New York: Truman Talley Books, St. Martin Press.

Entwistle, V., & O'Donnell, M. (2001). Evidence-based health care: What roles for patients. In A. Edwards & G. Elwyn (Eds.), *Evidence-Based Patient Choice.* New York: Oxford University Press.

Estabrooks, C. A. (1998). Will evidence-based practice make practice perfect? *Canadian Journal of Nursing, 30,* 15–36.

Fetterman, D. M., Kaftarian, S. J., & Wandersman, A. (1996). *Empowerment Evaluation: Knowledge & Tools for Self-Assessment & Accountability.* London: Sage.

Feuerbach, R. D., & Panniers, T. (2003). Building an expert system: Systematic approach to developing an instrument for data extraction from the literature. *Journal of Nursing Care Quality, 18*(2), 129–138.

Foxcroft, D. R., & Cole N. (2004). Organizational infrastructure to promote evidence-based nursing practice. *Cochrane Database of Systematic Reviews, 3.* Available at http://gateway.ut.ovid.com/gw1/ovidweb.cgi. Retrieved November 2, 2004.

Friere, P. (1970). *Pedagogy of the Oppressed.* New York: Seabury.

Funk, S. G., Tornquist, E. M., & Champagne, M. T. (1995). Barriers & facilitators of research utilization. *Nursing Clinics of North America, 30,* 395–407.

Greenwood, D., & Levin, M. (1998). *Introduction to Action Research: Social Research for Social Change.* Thousand Oaks, CA: Sage.

Habermas, J. (1985). *Theory of Communicative Action* (vol. 1). Boston: Beacon.

Higgs, J., Burn, A., & Jones, M. (2001). Integrating clinical reasoning and evidence-based practice. *AACN Clinical Issues: Advanced Practice in Acute and Critical Care, 12,* 482–490.

Institute of Medicine (IOM). (2003). Health professionals' education: A bridge to quality. Washington, DC: National Academy Press.

Johns, C., & Freshwater, D. (Eds.) (1998). *Transforming nursing through reflective practice.* London: Blackwell Science.

Lewin, K. (1946). Action research and minority problems. *Journal of Social Issues, 2*, 34–46.

McCleary, L., & Brown, G. (2003). Barriers to pediatric nurses' research utilization. *Journal of Advanced Nursing, 42*, 364–372.

Muir Gray, J. A. (2001). *Evidence-Based Health Care* (2nd ed.). London: Churchill Livingstone.

Newman, M., Papadopoulos, I., & Sigsworth, J. (1998). Barriers to evidence-based practice. *Clinical Effectiveness in Nursing, 2*, 11–20.

Nursing's Agenda for the Future: A call to the nation (2002). Washington, DC: The American Nurses Association, Inc. Available at www.NursingWorld.org/naf. Retrieved February 10, 2005.

Porter-O'Grady, T. (2003). Different age for leadership, Part 1: New context, new content. *Journal of Nursing Administration, 33*(2), 105–110.

Retsas, A. (2000). Barriers to using research evidence in nursing practice. *Journal of Advanced Nursing, 31*, 599–606.

Rogers, E. M. (1995). *Diffusion of Innovations* (4th ed.) New York: The Free Press.

Rutledge, D., Ropka, M., Greene, P., Nail, L., & Mooney, K. (1998). Barriers to research utilization for oncology staff nurses and nurse managers/clinical nurse specialists. *ONF, 25*, 497–506.

Sackett, D. L., Straus, S. E., Richardson, W. S., Rosenberg, W., & Haynes, R. B. (2000). *Evidence-Based Medicine: How to Practice and Teach EBM*. London: Churchill Livingstone.

Sanares, D., & Heliker, D. (2002). Implementation of an evidence-based nursing practice model: Disciplined Clinical Inquiry. *Journal for Nurses in Staff Development, 18*, 233–240.

Silva, M. C., Sorrell, J. M., & Sorrell, C. D. (1995). From Carper's patterns of knowing to ways of being: An ontological philosophical shift in nursing. *Advances in Nursing Science, 18*, 1–13.

Stetler, C. B. (2003). Role of the organization in translating research into evidence-based practice. *Outcomes Management, 7*(3), 97–103.

Stevens, K. (2001). Systematic reviews: The heart of evidence-based practice. *AACN Clinical Issues, 12*, 529–538.

Stringer, E. (1996). *Action Research: A Handbook for Practitioners*. Thousand Oaks, CA: Sage.

Stringer, E., & Genat, G. (2004). *Action Research in Health*. Upper Saddle River, NJ: Merrill, Prentice Hall.

Swan, B. A., & Boruch, R. F. (2004). Quality of evidence: Usefulness in measuring the quality of health care. *Medical Care, 42*(2), II-12–II-20.

Thompson, C., Cullum, N., McCaughan, D., Sheldon, T., & Raynor, P. (2004). Nurses, information use, and clinical decision making—the real world potential for evidence-based decisions in nursing. *Evidence-Based Nursing, 7*(3), 68–72.

Van Vlaenderen, H. (2001). Evaluating development programs: Building joint activity. *Evaluation and Program Planning, 24*, 343–352.

White, J. (1995). Patterns of knowing: Review, critique, and update. *Advances in Nursing Science, 17*(4), 73–86.

Wolf, F. M. (2000). Summarizing the evidence for clinical use. In J. P. Geyman, R. A. Deyo, & S. D. Ramsey (Eds), *Evidence-Based Clinical Practice: Concepts and Approaches*. Boston: Butterworth-Heinemann, 133–143.

CHAPTER 3

From Nursing Process to Nursing Synthesis: Evidence-Based Nursing Education

Marcia K. Flesner, Louise Miller,
Roxanne McDaniel, and Marilyn Rantz

Nursing education faces the daunting task of preparing registered nurses to participate in a health care environment where the pace of change is breathtaking. The explosion of research-based information and easier accessibility of the information leads to the expectation and responsibility of nursing staff to incorporate evidence-based knowledge into their practice setting. In addition, the practice sites available to nurses today range from the traditional hospital setting to home health and hospice, a multitude of specialty areas, and long-term care settings. The nurse as teacher is a major function of the profession in those settings, and the skills required to teach effectively are technical and difficult (Van Hoozer, Bratton, Ostmoe, Wienholtz, Craft, Albanese, & Gjerde, 1987). Today the practice environment for nurses is full of subordinate employees who perform delegated nursing functions that are the responsibilities of registered nurses, indicating a level of supervisory knowledge is essential for a registered nurse to possess.

Delivering a graduate nurse that possesses advanced skills as identified by Benner (1984) is an impossible task for nursing educators because expertise takes time to develop. But as Benner advised, "a strong educational preparation in the biological and psychosocial sciences and in nursing arts and science" (p.184) provides the basis for safe care and the background knowledge to ask the right questions. In the scientific age in which we live today, new medical advances are reported weekly, bombarding nurses with new information that can become overwhelming, regardless of the quality of the basic educational program. Graduation from nursing school is just the beginning of life-long learning that is essential to practice nursing competently and safely in the 21st century.

Since the 1970s, the nursing profession has been developing a scientific body of knowledge in the areas of nursing practice and nursing education (Polit &

Beck, 2003). As the body of knowledge grew, the nursing community became aware of the importance of scientific evidence needed for practice decisions. The communication of research findings started to become more available through the publication of journals devoted to nursing research. In the 1980s, the National Center for Nursing Research at the National Institutes of Health and the American Nurses Association Commission on Nursing Research were established to identify research priorities that focused on nursing practice.

In the 1990s, the development of clinical guidelines occurred as nursing specialty groups, the American Nurses Association, and the federal government responded to nurses' need for timely information for effective decision-making. The Agency for Healthcare Research and Quality (formerly the Agency for Health Care Policy and Research) established 12 Evidence-Based Practice Centers in 1997 (Agency for Healthcare Research and Quality, 2004). These centers develop evidence reports and technology assessments on topics of clinical importance to health care organizations, and a thirteenth evidence-based center was added in 2002. A brief listing of topics being investigated of interest to nursing are: blood pressure monitoring; practice outside the clinic area; end-of-life care; best strategies for quality improvement; management of cancer associated pain and related symptoms; and rehabilitation for traumatic brain injury.

Today, nurses can access research-based clinical information that provides guidance for clinical practice via a variety of media, including publications, journals, and Web sites. The educational preparation of registered nurses has responded to the proliferation of research findings since the 1970s by the addition of a research component of curricula in the undergraduate-nursing curriculum, and by focusing on preparing master-level nurses to conduct nursing research (Polit & Beck, 2003). Inclusion of informatics in nursing education programs has also been a direct consequence of the rapidly changing health care environment.

The Institute of Medicine (IOM), Committee on Quality of Health Care in America, published the pivotal report, *Crossing the Quality Chasm* (2001), which, in part, addresses the notion of evidence-based practice. The report uses the following definition of evidence-based practice adapted from Sackett, Straus, Richardson, Rosenberg, and Haynes (2000).

> Evidence-based practice is the integration of best research evidence with clinical expertise and patient values. Best research evidence refers to clinically relevant research, often from the basic health and medical sciences, but especially from patient-centered clinical research into the accuracy and precision of diagnostic tests (including the clinical examination); the power of prognostic markers; and the efficacy and safety of therapeutic, rehabilitative, and preventative regimens. Clinical expertise means the ability to use clinical skills and past experience to rapidly identify each patient's unique health state and diagnosis, individual risks and benefits of potential interventions, and personal values and expectations. Patient val-

ues refer to the unique preferences, concerns, and expectations that each patient brings to a clinical encounter and that must be integrated into clinical decisions if they are to serve the patient (Institute of Medicine, 2001, p. 147).

The rapid evolution of evidence-based practice, first in medicine and then other health fields, is influencing the design of nursing education programs of today and the future. The goal of this chapter is to discuss educational changes that should be considered by nurse educators, so that nursing educational programs can respond to the changing fields where registered nurses will practice.

HISTORY OF EVIDENCE-BASED MEDICINE AND PRACTICE

Since the 1970s, American nurses and physicians have developed and focused on evidence-based medicine (EBM) and evidence-based practices (Titler et al., 2001), especially as medical advances have proliferated at a pace that few professionals maintain. In addition, American consumers became better informed with subsequent growing expectations that their health care providers would make recommendations on the best available scientific information. The opinions and intuition of nurses and physicians could no longer be as reliable as the latest systemic review of high quality research.

Nursing practice and education have been influenced by the use of research in nursing practice. As more nurses with masters and doctoral level education entered the work force in the last 30 years, the research-based data produced by their scientific investigation acknowledged the integral role that nursing plays in health care (Polit & Beck, 2003). The National Center for Nursing Research at the National Institutes of Health and the American Nurses Association Cabinet on Nursing Research have promoted and provided guidance by focusing research on nursing practice and education issues.

Archie Cochrane, a British physician, is associated with the movement of EBM (Reynolds, 2000). Cochrane believed that because health resources are always limited, resources used to deliver services to patients need to be shown to be effective. From his personal physician–patient experiences, Cochrane described the problems associated with applying research principles to the field of health care as well as the difficulties of using research trials for individual patient care. To integrate research with medical practice, he advocated use of randomized clinical trials for evaluating treatment methods, and pioneered the use of systematic reviews and meta-analyses in medicine.

In 1989, a British medical group, headed by Murray Enkin, published a review of the 'evidence' for effective care in pregnancy and childbirth (Enkin, Keirse, & Chalmers, 1989). This landmark work helped articulate the need for other health care professionals, particularly physicians, to systematically collate best practice information from research reports and make practice decisions based on the collective results.

Paralleling the developments in the United Kingdom, faculty at McMaster University in Canada, who had pioneered problem-based, self-directed learning, integrated the application of research findings into medical education (Reynolds, 2000). Central to this approach was the integration of clinical practice with research and use of research methods to make patient care decisions (diagnosis, treatment/therapy, and prognosis). This approach was named evidence-based medicine in 1992 by a group at McMaster's (Sackett et al., 2000).

The British and Canadian movements in EBM led to the development of databases for systematic reviews, meta-analyses, clinical guidelines, and best practices, such as The Cochrane Library (http://www.concrane.co.uk), the Best Evidence Database (http://www.evidence-basedmedicine.com), and Bandolier (http://www.jr2.ox.ac.uk/Bandolier).

Development of computer technology and the Internet has also influenced the evolution of evidence-based practice in health care settings. The ability of computers to process large databases, retain historical records, and speedily access information has led to computerized clinical charting systems. The Internet has allowed health care professionals to access up-to-date research information and clinical guidelines based on systematic literature reviews, irrespective of their location. Nurses will see nursing practice change on a regular basis as more evidence-based information is produced by nurse researchers.

In addition, the "gold standard" for evidence, which traditionally has been randomized clinical trials, has been broadened to include other types of systematically acquired information. These include other types of epidemiologic research as well as patient interviews, patient surveys, and data gathered using other qualitative methods.

Muir Gray (2001) identified four common factors that impact health care delivery globally:

- Increasing health care expenditures
- The inability of countries to pay for all the services demanded by professionals and patients
- Variation in the rates of delivery of health services within a country and among countries
- Delayed implementation of research findings into practice.

One response to the challenges faced by health care organizations and health care providers has been the movement to evidence-based approach to the delivery of care. From the research studies done and systematic reviews performed of those studies, the body of clinical knowledge has grown over the years, with best practice guidelines and treatment protocols emerging (Roberts & Yeager, 2004). Evidence-based nursing practice results when nurses use the latest scientific evidence in their practice, targeting patient outcomes and best practice interventions.

STATUS OF NURSING EDUCATION

Formal nursing education in the United States began as hospital training programs that were under the direction and supervision of physicians. The main purpose of these schools was to prepare nurses to perform skills necessary to care for hospitalized patients and to carry out physicians' orders (Kalisch & Kalisch, 1987). In hospital-based training schools, education was an apprenticeship where students were responsible for staffing the hospitals, with most of their time devoted to working on the wards. Students learned by providing service to the patients in the hospital, with little or no formal class work. Their "education" was based on ritual and tradition.

In 1893, the first organization for developing standards of nursing education was formed. The organization became the National League for Nursing and established the first standard nursing education curriculum in 1917. This curriculum provided the outline for the three-year diploma program. It was highly prescriptive and did not allow for diversity in education. In 1937, the guidelines were revised and named A Curriculum Guide for Schools of Nursing.

In the early 1900s, nursing education moved into a collegiate setting. Many of the early university programs were five-year programs. These programs initially prepared students to be nurse educators. In 1908, the American Hospital Association urged a return to the earlier educational practice of two-year courses to meet the increasing demand for nurses to staff the numerous hospitals that were opening throughout the country.

Nursing education was also influenced by major military conflicts. During World War I and immediately afterwards, there was a marked increase in the demand for nurses. To meet this demand, admission and training standards were lowered. A committee, funded by the Rockefeller Foundation to study the education programs of nurses, published a report that recommended higher standards of education, special training for instructors, stronger associations with colleges and universities, and adequate financial support for nursing education programs.

World War II also brought about an increased demand for trained nurses. Once again, a committee was formed to study nursing education, but this time it was composed of representatives of the major nursing organizations. In 1948, the committee published the Brown Report with major recommendations for nursing. These recommendations included: accreditation of schools, standards for faculty preparation, improved courses in hospital-based schools, and more utilization of university teaching resources. It also recommended using the term "professional" to designate those who studied in an accredited professional school and to establish two-year college-based programs to help relieve the shortage of qualified nurses. Following this report, the number of baccalaureate programs steadily increased.

The associate degree education program was started in 1952, based on a research project by Mildred Montag. The associate degree nurse (ADN) was to be a bedside nurse or a "technical nurse." The ADN's education was originally based in community and junior colleges and could be completed in two years. Montag envisioned the ADN graduate to be a technician with a narrower scope of practice than the professional nurse. The education of the ADN included general education along with nursing content. These programs were not intended to include leadership and management or research, but focused on preparing the nurse to work under the guidance of a professional nurse. The original vision of the technical or associate nurse did not include integrating research into practice. According to the American Nurses Association (1965), the education of the ADN was to be scientifically based, but technically oriented, and not concerned with developing theory.

Over the years, the idea of an associate degree in nursing as a terminal degree has changed. Articulation agreements with baccalaureate nursing programs are common throughout the country. Although ADNs comprise 52% of nursing graduates, they are only 40% of the RN workforce (U.S. Department of Health and Human Services, 2000).

The first graduate program in nursing was established at Columbia University's Teachers College. This master's level program was to prepare nurses for the roles of educator or administrator. These roles dominated nursing master's education until the development of advanced practice roles, such as the clinical nurse specialist and nurse practitioner. Currently, almost 85% of the students enrolled in masters programs are learning these advanced practice roles (American Association of Colleges of Nursing, 2003). The curriculum of the master's program varies depending upon the area of specialization, but should include core content for all advanced practice nurses. The content areas for core competencies include: research, health care policy, ethics, role, theory, diversity and social issues, and health promotion and disease prevention (American Association of Colleges of Nursing, 1996). Because educational preparation and research experience include these core competencies, the master's prepared nurse is able to provide leadership in evidence-based nursing practice. The course work in research, theory, and specialty content areas allows advanced practice nurses to critically examine the research data and to use the latest scientific evidence in their practice.

Baccalaureate and master's nursing education continue to respond to the demand for evidence-based practice. The skills needed for registered nurses to practice in an evidence-based work environment will continue to place demands on nursing educators. The teaching methods and traditions of clinical nursing education are no longer sufficient to meet the needs of future registered nurses. Recommended skills needed for evidence-based practice follow.

SKILLS NECESSARY FOR EVIDENCE-BASED PRACTICE

Critical Thinking Skills

"Critical thinking is defined . . . as the rational examination of ideas, inferences, assumptions, principles, arguments, conclusions, issues, statements, beliefs and action" (Bandman & Bandman, 1995, p. 7). Alfaro-LeFevre (1999) advised that if we want to survive and thrive, we need to think critically. Critical thinking is an essential skill that student nurses must develop during their educational program. Purposeful and goal-directed thinking is needed to manage and direct the nursing care of people with chronic and complex diseases.

Pesut and Herman (1999) reviewed the evolution of nursing process that had provided the structure for thinking in nursing since the 1950s. The four-step model of nursing process (assessment, planning, intervention, and evaluation) was an important development in clinical nursing, as it forced nurses to think before acting when providing care to patients. As the profession gained information on nursing care problems over the next 20 years using the model, a need was identified to classify and standardize the nomenclature used to describe commonly occurring problems. Work began in 1973 on the development of nursing diagnosis at the first Nursing Diagnosis Conference.

The second phase of the nursing process evolution identified by Pesut and Herman started in 1973 when the American Nurses Association expanded the model to five steps: assessment, diagnosis, planning, implementation, and evaluation. As researchers gathered information about processes and products of diagnostic reasoning in the 1980s, the complexity involved in information gathering and decision-making by nurses became apparent. The advantages and disadvantages of the nursing process were debated by the profession, as problem identification and solving were now being identified as hypothesis formulation and testing. Benner (1984) showed that thinking occurred differently among nurses, based on the experiences they had gained and that intuition was another element of decision-making.

Pesut and Herman developed what they called the third generation nursing process. Titled the Outcome-Present State-Test (OPT) Model of Reflective Clinical Reasoning, OPT is a new model of reasoning that provides for a structure of iterative reasoning. New models of reasoning are needed in the current outcomes-focused health care environment. The OPT model uses the North America Nursing Diagnosis Association, Nursing Intervention Classification, and Nursing Outcome Classification taxonomies, which provide a vocabulary for clinical reasoning. Three worksheets (The OPT Model, The Clinical Reasoning Web, and The Thinking Strategies) are used to determine the focus of care for patients. Another component of OPT is reflection, where the nurses review their reasoning to discover flaws in their thinking. As the evolution of the nursing process continues, nursing faculty will need to continue their education on the developing models, so that future nurses have had exposure to the latest approach to clinical reasoning before entering their practice.

Nursing educators can no longer focus on mastery of skills and content to prepare nurses for jobs in the future. Completion of 10-page care plans will not prepare students to provide skilled care based on evidence-based knowledge. Research in the fields of critical thinking and nursing education revealed a mixed bag of results, but have raised concerns about the ability of current curriculums to foster development of critical thinking in students (Krichbaum, Lewis, & Duckett, 1997).

Figure 3.1 is an example of a critical thinking exercise used at the Sinclair School of Nursing at the University of Missouri-Columbia, Sinclair School of Nursing.

Figure 3.1   An Example of a Critical Thinking Exercise for Nursing Students

Implementing Evidence in Clinical Practice

Decision Theory

The first considerations are to determine what options we should consider, and how we go about making that decision. We will use *Decision Theory* from operations management in business to analyze the thinking behind a decision "to or not to" implement. In our example, we will use decision theory to make a clinical judgment to, or not to, pop a blister.

Decision theory is a method for exploring possible outcomes. To use this strategy, the first step is to generate a list of possible outcomes. After the list is established, outcomes can be enhanced by assigning probabilities, or asking the question, "how likely will one outcome occur compared to another outcome?" Use the diagram to outline our example, deciding whether or not to pop a blister. We ask the initial question, "if you pop a blister, what is the likelihood that it will become infected?" You will agree that if you intentionally pop a blister, there is a chance that it will become infected, and a chance that it will not become infected.

Figure 3.1 An Example of a Critical Thinking Exercise for Nursing Students (*continued*)

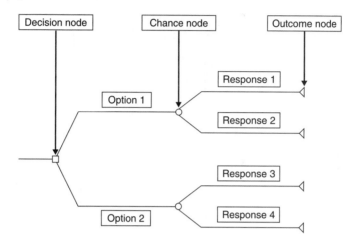

From Earlam, S., Brecker, N., & Vaughan, B. (2000). *Cascading Evidence*. Hong Kong: Adis International.

Question 1 in the decision tree is, "should you or should you not pop the blister?" The decision may not be 100% clear in your mind, because your nursing background has taught you that there are considerations for popping it and not popping it. The point at which you decide whether you should or should not pop the blister is called a "decision node." The decision node separates option 1 (yes – pop the blister) from option 2 (no – don't pop the blister).

Both option 1 and option 2 have a chance that the blister will become infected and not become infected. This decision point is called the "chance node." The chance node brings about response 1 or 2 (infected or not infected) for option 1. Option 2 has the same range of responses.

The outcomes nodes are either health recovery or chronic infection. We now have reached the point where we created a conceptual scheme to explore the possible outcomes. You now ask yourself if you have really answered the question whether or not to pop the blister. Actually, what you have done is listed as a set of outcomes as shown in the decision tree. Of the listed outcomes, what is most likely to happen?

We can also use our decision tree to determine the most likely outcome by assigning probabilities at each node. The decision node, whether to pop the blister or not, is really not a 50–50 decision, because of the chance of accidental popping. An accidental pop makes the probability of option 1 60%, and therefore the probability of option 2 is 40%. At the chance node for this revised example (accidental popping), assign a probability of infected versus not infected. In my experience, a popped blister becomes infected only 20% of the time.

Figure 3.1   An Example of a Critical Thinking Exercise for Nursing Students (*continued*)

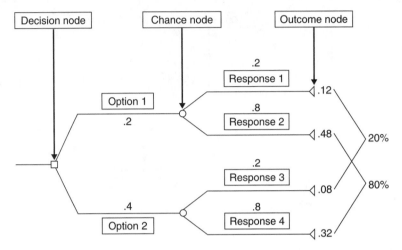

Now that we have added these sets of probabilities to our decision tree, we can estimate the probability of each of the four possible responses. You can then calculate the probability of the outcome.

Prior to assigning probabilities, you may have guessed that the chance of a blister becoming infected was less than 50%, but you may not have known exactly how much less than 50%. By assigning probabilities, the chance is actually 20% (not simply less than 50%) as we have demonstrated in our decision tree.

There are key assumptions in this analysis:

- A correct and complete list of responses was generated;
- The correct probability values were chosen;
- All possible outcomes were generated and addressed.

We stopped at the outcome node of infection. We could "peel back the onion" and ask once again about the possibility (probability) of the infection becoming mild, moderate, or chronic. So you have a choice at the outcome node to continue to explore the impact of additional decisions and interventions (e.g., antibiotic treatment with [a] multiple choices of antibiotics and [b] various outcomes from antibiotics), or additional outcomes by way of the chance nodes (e.g., superficial vs. deep infection). Or to expand the decision tree even further, you can combine both decision and chance nodes to further explore a larger family of outcomes.

A decision tree is used to provide precision to the likely outcome for the decision with which you are faced. Consider the excruciating detail we outlined for a fairly simple decision whether or not to pop a blister.

Exposure to Research Knowledge

Baccalaureate nursing programs require research as a component of the nursing curriculum. The goal of a research course is to introduce nursing students to the basics of the scientific approach of research in the belief that they will be able to use the information produced to provide guidance to their nursing practice upon graduation. It is challenging to convince a room full of busy students who are eager to learn clinical skills that nursing research can assist them to be proficient nurses in the future. The language, scientific concepts, constructs, and theories of research can be a challenge, and if there is not a connection made between their clinical and classroom experiences, any knowledge from the course may soon be shelved in the part of the brain labeled "rarely used."

To improve the use of research knowledge by baccalaureate students, nursing research should be integrated into the curriculum of nursing programs. Wheeler, Fasano, and Burr (1995) surveyed National League for Nursing programs and found that none of the 67 respondents reported integrating research into the curriculum. An example of integrating research into one course was provided by Kenty (2001). Named the Collaborative Learning Project (CLP), an adult health course was "designed to increase student's research knowledge and change attitudes, but more importantly to help students understand the importance of evidence-based practice" (p. 182).

Kenty designed CLP to follow the five research-related functions proposed by the American Nurses Association in 1989: "(1) identify a practice problem; (2) interpret and evaluate the applicability of specific practice problem; (3) implement the practice innovation; (4) evaluate the practice innovation; (4) evaluate the practice innovation using measuring outcomes; and (5) share research findings in an oral presentation" (p. 182). Evaluation of the project revealed significantly increased research knowledge in students who participated in CLP when compared to students who did not participate. Positive changes in the students' attitudes were also reported, with students demonstrating synthesis of research concepts.

Assisting students to critically examine research results is a basic skill needed for evidence-based practice. Figure 3.2 is an example of a worksheet used in a master's course at the University of Missouri-Columbia, Sinclair School of Nursing. Students who use the worksheet are able to demonstrate their ability to understand research designs used to answer clinical questions.

Integrating research into practice-based experiences needs the commitment of faculty and clinical sponsors, which will require development of collaborative relationships between the two groups. Practice setting issues will arise as discussed by Kenty, but through planning and postevaluation with staff of the clinical site, the difficulties can be reduced or avoided. Integrating research into the

Figure 3.2   Evidence-Based Practice Worksheet Used at University of Missouri-Columbia

Evidence-Based Practice Worksheet

To critique your article, answer the following questions. Be sure that you critique your article, not simply summarize the information presented in the article. To critique, you make judgments of clarity, appropriateness, accuracy, and reliability of the components of the study. Begin the paper with a title page, listing the citation, i.e., title of the article, authors, and journal information. You need to include sections on purpose/goal/hypothesis of the study, groups studied (sample), how the study was conducted (methods, tools used, how data were collected), results and conclusions, and of course, 'so what', i.e., significance of the study, or said another way, 'what difference did this study make in the whole scheme of things?' The information in italics under each point is discussion points to include in your critique.

Purpose

1. Choose some phrases from the abstract or first paragraphs that tell you what the study is about. *Restate the question—don't copy it from the article.*
2. Look at the information about the authors. Where are they from? What is their education and practice area, e.g., medicine, nursing, epidemiology, psychology, etc.? *How does their area of expertise affect the choice of the study question and how the question is asked?*
3. Does it appear to be a relevant question? For example, is this question one that needs to be answered? Is there a need for more information about this in the practice world? Is this type of information already available? If so, is that information conflicting and does it need clarification, or does this study reinforce what is already known? *Sort out the answers to these questions, and emphasize the strengths and/or weaknesses of the overall purpose.*
4. Is there background information (other studies) included? Does it give you an idea of what is already known (or not known) about this particular issue? Does it lead you right into this current study, i.e., does it 'make the case' for doing this study? Is it clearly written? Are there some omissions about this issue that should have been included to better understand why these authors chose to do this study? Does the background information seem skewed (or twisted) from what is known about this issue? In other words, have they been selective about what information they have included just to prove a point? *Make a judgment about all of these and include a statement about the relevance of the background information and the relationship/importance to the current study question.*

Sample and Groups Studied

5. Who is being studied? Describe the groups, e.g., by gender, by race/ethnic group, etc. and by number of people included in the study. Now, forget about who the authors picked to study—Think about who should be included to really understand the research question and make the results relevant.

Figure 3.2   Evidence-Based Practice Worksheet Used at University of Missouri-Columbia *(continued)*

Compare the kinds of people you <u>think</u> should be included to the ones who <u>were</u> included. *Who are omitted in the study that you included? Why are they important? How could the authors have included them, or could they? What potential information would these "omitted" people add?*

6. Is there a statement about protection of patient's rights? Things to consider include:

   (1) were participants informed of the study prior to participation?

   (2) were participants informed that they could drop out at any time?

   (3) were notes, interview transcripts, patient records, and the like protected from access to others and chance of 'falling into the wrong hands'?

   (4) was patient information coded with numbers or other symbols that detached the patient's name from the information?

   (5) was the coded number system with patient names kept separate from the actual patient information (patient data)?

   (6) do the results have the potential of jeopardizing the health and well-being of the subjects?

   (Note: All credible research must be approved by Institutional Review Boards (also known as IRBs). These boards protect the rights of human subjects. These boards came about as a result of the Nazi atrocities committed against the Jews, the Tuskegee experiments, and other horrible human experiments. It is important that patients who participate in research are informed of their rights. On the other hand, requirements for patient consent also can pose some significant methodological issues for researchers, such as seeking out vulnerable groups who may be viewed as exploited subjects in research.) *Look for a statement in the article about the participants receiving informed consent and/or approval by the IRB.*

Study Design and Methods for Collecting Patient Data

7. How was this study designed? Is it one group, or were the participants divided into two groups? Did the authors pick a readily accessible group to study (also known as convenience sample)? Or did the authors work hard to make it a random group? A random group means that everyone who has a possibility of participating has a chance to participate. For example, when studying people in the state of Missouri, everyone has equal chance to participate. So, *how many groups were included in this study? One, two, or more?* Should economic impact be considered as a component of the study? *Were economic impact data included as a dimension of the study design? If not, should they have been, and how should the questions about costs have been asked?*

8. Was there an intervention done in this study? This is common with more than one group, i.e., one group receives a 'treatment' and the other receives no treatment. Or was this study descriptive, meaning that the data describe or 'tell a story' about the people studied? *Determine if the study is descrip-*

Figure 3.2   Evidence-Based Practice Worksheet Used at University of Missouri-Columbia *(continued)*

tive or includes an intervention/treatment. If you are familiar with types of epidemiological studies, e.g., prevalence or cross-sectional, case control, and clinical trials, *specify the type.*

9. What methods did the authors use to collect information? Did they interview the participants? Did they survey the participants? Did they use patient records? Did they use other methods to collect information? Did they use a combination of methods, e.g., interviews plus patient records? Did they give you a sample of the questions asked and/or the information (variables) collected? Did they use a standardized tool, e.g., BP cuff, repeatedly used questionnaire, etc? Were these tools checked out to make sure they give the same answers over and over (also called 'reliability')? Was the procedure (the step-by-step) for collecting the patient information explained in the article? Do you have a good idea of how this information was collected? Could you do it again using the description given by the authors? *Think about what information you think should be collected to answer the question (see #1). Did the authors collect the 'right' information? What other questions should have been asked? How could you get that information? In your lesson instruction, this is explained as 'outcomes' (item #5 in your list).

Results, Conclusions, and 'So What'

10. Results and conclusions are different. Results are a listing of compiled data that has been analyzed. For example, data can be reported as statistics, as summary statements, and/or in tables. Conclusions are the next step beyond results. *Conclusions represent judgments made by the authors about the significance of the results, applicability to the group(s) studied, and relevance to the research question.* Again, refer to your lesson instruction, item #6, for other ways to ask these questions. In your judgment, *do the data reflect the conclusions the authors draw, or are they jumping to conclusions that should not be made? Are there alternative explanations for the data? What are those alternative explanations? Do the authors suggest alternative explanations?*

11. Finally, 'so what'. *Does this study make a difference? Can you see its implications to a broader group of people? Does it make you think of more questions that should be asked about the problem/issue? What should the next steps be for this problem/issue? Is there an expression of economic impact, if appropriate to the research study?*

From the online policy course of the Sinclair School of Nursing at the University of Missouri-Columbia. Reprinted with permission.

course work of a nursing program also requires a commitment by the nursing program leader and faculty members. The transition will require additional work initially, but students who participate in such a nursing program will be prepared for evidence-based practice.

Information Technology Knowledge and Skills

Students who enter college today are expected to have gained essential skills in the use of computers and software. Nursing students will use computerized information systems (IS) at their clinical sites throughout their nursing program. They must be prepared to handle different IS if they are to enter data correctly and efficiently. Patient and clinical encounters at all levels take place for the purpose of gathering and exchanging information that can be shared with other clinicians. Unfortunately, there is no uniform method of collecting data in the health care delivery system. Due to the lack of a uniform data collection method, nursing educators are challenged to prepare students to work in health care systems where timely information sharing is needed, but a common nursing technology system does not exist as a base for nursing informatics programs.

Nursing educators must develop the skills necessary to include information technology content in their nursing curriculum and be able to teach the content, so that nursing students are skilled upon graduation. Research by McNeil and colleagues (2003) revealed that, of the faculty teaching information technology in 166 baccalaureate and higher nursing degree programs, 39% of faculty were rated at the advanced beginner's level and 18% reported their faculty at the novice level. The information skills of nursing faculty need to advance beyond those levels if students are to be prepared upon graduation with a level of competence that is needed for evidence-based practice skills.

Clinical-decision support systems (CDSS) are software that integrates information on the patient with a computer knowledge base (Institute of Medicine, 2001). The goal of CDSS is to assist health care providers in making clinical decisions. Although development and evaluation of CDSS has had minimal impact on health care delivery systems, the 2001 IOM report advised that future systems potentially will enhance evidence-based practice. Nurses who are prepared to be computer proficient and capable of using new CDSS will be able to adapt to a rapidly evolving technology scene in the future, where handheld computers may become the norm in the work setting.

Information Literacy

Information literacy has been described as a prerequisite to evidence-based nursing practice (Shorten, Wallace, & Crookes, 2001). Information literacy means that a nurse is able to recognize when information is needed to plan and provide nursing care, and has the ability to find, evaluate, and effectively use the information (American Library Association, 2001). For nursing students to become information literate, the skill of locating relevant clinical information should be incorporated into nursing curriculums.

Educators in Australia described such a curriculum-integrated model in several publications (Shorten, Wallace, & Crookes, 2001; Wallace, Shorten, Crookes, McGurk & Brewer, 1999; Wallace, Shorten, & Russell, 1997). An interdisciplinary partnership between a faculty librarian and nursing faculty led to the development of library-based learning activities and complementary assessment tasks that were integrated into a fundamental clinical nursing subject. The program was structured to ensure successful searching of the library's electronic databases, which improved student self-confidence, and contributed to student motivation and skill development. Evaluation of the model provided statistically significant evidence that students who participated in the program were successful in developing information literacy skills and retention of the skills at the end of the study. Nursing faculty members are encouraged to review the experiences referenced above for guidance when working to design educational programs to develop information literacy skills in nursing students.

Role Modeling by Faculty

Nursing faculty are the first nurses who have an opportunity to influence nursing students. Initially, students learn through classroom experience, reading assignments, and interactions with faculty and other students. Faculty members are the key role models for student nurses throughout their educational program, and they influence how students learn and retain knowledge. It is no longer acceptable to ask students to memorize data about a clinical topic and then to test on the memorized data. Application of the knowledge in a clinical setting should be the goal. Critical thinking can and must be taught, and nursing faculty need to be experts on the topic of critical thinking development.

At the undergraduate level, innovative approaches will be needed to develop learning experiences that promote outcome-oriented thinking. Alfaro-LeFevre (1999) offered critical thinking exercises and nursing research exercises at the end of each chapter in her book to assist nurses to improve thinking skills, expanding beyond good problem solving to reflective thinking. Critical thinking is described succinctly as "a commitment to look for the best way, based on the most current research and practice findings" (p. 59). Faculty must assist novice learners to progress through the steps of learning how to think critically. As they mentor students, they need to interweave evidence-based data into the curriculum and learning experiences of the nursing program and the clinical setting.

Nursing faculty must also role model the value of nursing research in the clinical setting. In addition to learning the basic concepts of research, students need to learn how to apply those research findings into a practice setting. Several strategies can be used to actively engage students in research. One strategy to involve students in the process is to use a research proposal to demonstrate the principles of the research process and involve students in the data collection and analysis. Another strategy is to have students provide the data for a research study. Demographic data can be collected about the students and then used to compare to previous classes and the literature.

One way to teach evidence-based practice in a research course is to put students in small groups and provide them with research articles to critique. The students share their critiques and then compare the studies to clinical settings where the findings could be implemented. The next step is to discuss if the findings are ready for use or if additional research is needed. If the research could be implemented, the students discuss how to put the research findings into practice and how to evaluate the implementation. Actively engaging undergraduate students in the research process increases understanding and appreciation of the importance of research for evidence-based practice.

The importance of evidence-based practice in nursing is highlighted by the proposal for the master's prepared clinical nurse leader that has been put forth by the American Association of Colleges of Nursing. Evidence-based practice is identified as an essential curriculum element with identified competencies and clinical experiences.

Selecting an evidence-based practice model for use in a nursing program will be a necessary challenge. Mohide and King (2003) reported locating 23 distinct evidence-based practice models in a literature search of several databases. The evolution of four evidence-based practice models was reviewed by Pape (2003) and included: Iowa Model of Research-Based Practice to Promote Quality Care, Stetler Model, Rogers Model, and The Academic Center for Evidence-Based Practice (ACE) Star Model. The Iowa Model was developed in 1994 to be used as a guide for nursing staff to use research findings to improve patient care (Titler et al., 2001). Revisions have been made to the Iowa model based on feedback from users and prompted by changes in the health care market. The Stetler Model, first reported on in 1976, and refined and expanded in 1994, consists of six phases to use at the practitioner level to apply research finds to practice (Stetler, 1994).

The Rogers Model consists of five stages: knowledge, persuasion, decision, implementation, and confirmation (Burns & Grove, 1999). The ACE Model, developed by the University of Texas Health Science Center at San Antonio, consists of five knowledge transformation steps, which are represented by five points on the ACE Star Model. The ACE Model framework organizes evidence-based practice processes and approaches, revealing the relationships between the five steps. The University also is a funded ACE, and information on its funded studies can be located at http://www.acestar.uthscsa.edu/. Faculty members need to familiarize themselves with the evolving models and integrate a model into their curriculum. Models help to clarify and visualize the process for students.

Finally, nursing faculty need to be cognizant of the differences between novice thinking and expert thinking. Faculty have experiences and expanded knowledge that allows them to generate better hypotheses when problem solving with a patient situation. Novice students are eager to act before assessing and have limited knowledge. Learning about evidence-based practice can occur when faculty are supportive and knowledgeable about how critical thinking is taught.

Communication Skills

The availability of evidence-based practice guidelines does not guarantee that practicing nurses will use them. As nursing graduates enter the work force, they will be confronted with a work force encrusted in the practice models of the institution. As we know, many nursing practices are not based on facts, but on routines and traditions of the institution. Graduates should be prepared to be greeted with resistance from co-workers who may have had minimal exposure to research principles or had minimal opportunity to develop critical thinking skills. It is easier to do a job when you just follow the rules instead of analyzing each situation and do what is appropriate for each individual patient.

Graduate nurses will need to be effective and skilled communicators when introducing evidence-based practice information in their work setting. They will need skills for working with groups, managing change, and disseminating information. The first year of nursing practice is a difficult time for recent graduates, and the challenge of introducing a new approach of problem solving while developing their clinical skills only adds to the stress and anxiety levels of the individual.

Understanding why nurses resist technology is important knowledge for graduate nurses to have. Introduction of evidence-based practice information can be unsettling for nursing staff. A common fear among practicing nurses is that obtaining the needed information will be time-consuming, and there is little time available in a work setting where nurses are already overloaded. Being an advocate for evidence-based practice is a challenging endeavor if the nurse is not prepared to communicate and advocate on behalf of evidence-based practices within the work setting and among team members.

Educational Preparation

Nurses who graduate from baccalaureate nursing programs are knowledgeable about basic research methods and principles. The authors believe nursing graduates who participate in educational programs at the collegiate level are the nurses who will be prepared to practice in an evidence-based practice environment.

Pape (2003) advocates on behalf of the role of knowledge broker when implementing evidence-based nursing practice. The knowledge broker is viewed as the change agent who can facilitate a team to collaborate toward a common goal. Masters-prepared nurses are ideal for the role of knowledge broker. Their advanced education, specialization in a clinical area, and research participation at the collegiate level have prepared them for evidence-based practice.

FUTURE CHALLENGES

Nursing educators face numerous challenges to adapt nursing programs with the same pace that occurs in the real world. Learning transmission increasingly occurs by electronic communication methods, and this transition is changing the way nursing education is delivered. Rapid change can be scary, but it can also be a time of wonderful growth, if individuals are willing to be risk takers. The ability and willingness to work with the new technology of today and the future allows those risk takers to help design the new structure of nursing education. The teaching of evidence-based practice in nursing programs is but one of many innovations that faculty will use to prepare future nurses to close the gap between research and practice.

Practicing health care from an evidence base has become necessary as more information is generated and available via rapid access technology. To adequately prepare future nurses to perform their jobs, educators must offer educational opportunities to explore and use various data sources and technologies that will become routine and mandatory in the worksite. Nurses will need critical thinking and decision-making skills as they implement "evidence" in practice, considering whether, for example, a guideline is appropriate or a prescribed treatment is supported by most current research practice. These skills are best taught while in school, in simulated situations, where discussion can occur, options can be considered, and outcomes evaluated. This can be accomplished by assignments such as structured critiques of research articles, with follow-up application of findings and implications to clinical practice situations.

REFERENCES

Alfaro-LeFevre, R. (1999). *Critical Thinking in Nursing: A Practical Approach* (2nd ed.). Philadelphia: W. B. Saunders.

American Association of Colleges of Nursing. (1996). *The Essentials of Master's Education for Advanced Practice Nursing.* Washington, DC: Author.

American Association of Colleges of Nursing. (2003). *Enrollment and Graduations in Baccalaureate and Graduate Programs in Nursing,* 2003–2004. Washington, DC: AACN.

American Library Association. Objectives for Information Literacy Instruction: A Model Statement for Academic Librarians. Available at http://www.ala.org/ala/acrl/acrlstandards/objectivesinformation.htm. Accessed September 1, 2004.

American Nurses Association. (1965). *Position Paper on Education.* Kansas City, MO: American Nurses Association.

American Nurses Association. (1989). *Education for participating in research.* Kansas City, MO: American Nurses Association.

Bandman, E. L., & Bandman, B. (1995). *Critical Thinking in Nursing* (2nd ed.). Stanford, CT: Appleton.

Benner, P. (2001). *From Novice to Expert.* Upper Saddle River, NJ: Prentice Hall.

Burns, N., & Grove, S. K. (1999). *Understanding Nursing Research* (2nd ed.). Philadelphia: W. B. Saunders.

Earlam, S., Brecker, N., & Vaughan, B. (2000). *Cascading Evidence.* Hong Kong: Adis International.

Enkin, M., Keirse, M. J. N. C., & Chalmers, I. (1989). *A Guide to Effective Care in Pregnancy and Childbirth.* Oxford, UK: Oxford University Press.

Institute of Medicine. (2001). *Crossing the Quality Chasm: A New Health System for the 21st Century.* Washington, DC: National Academy Press.

Kalisch, P., & Kalisch, B. (1987). *The Challenging Image of the Nurse.* Lebanon, IN: Addison-Wesley.

Kenty, J. R. (2001). Weaving undergraduate research into practice-based experiences. *Nursing Educator, 26*(4), 182–186.

Krichbaum, K., Lewis, M., & Duckett, L. (1997). Critical thinking: What is it and how do we teach it? In J. C. McClosky & H. K. Grace (Eds.), *Current Issues in Nursing* (5th ed.). St. Louis, MO: C. V. Mosby, pp. 169–179.

McNeil, B. J., Elfrink, V. L., Bickford, C. J., Pierce, S. T., Beyea, S. C., Averill, C., & Klappenbach, C. (2003). Nursing information technology knowledge, skills and preparation of student nurses, faculty, and clinicians: A U.S. Survey. *Journal of Nursing Education, 42*(8), 341–348.

Mohide, E. A. & King, B. (2003). Building a foundation for evidence-based practice: Experiences in a tertiary hospital. *Evidence-Based Nursing, 6*(4):100–103.

Muir Gray, J. A. (2001). *Evidence-Based Healthcare* (2nd ed.). Edinburgh, UK: Churchill Livingstone.

Pape, T. M. (2003). Evidence-based nursing practice: To infinity and beyond. *The Journal of Continuing Education in Nursing, 34*(4), 154–161.

Pesut, D. J., & Herman, J. (1999). *Clinical Reasoning: The Art & Science of Critical & Creative Thinking*. Albany, NY: Delmar Publishers.

Polit, D. F., & Beck, C. T. (2003). *Nursing Research: Principles and Methods*. Philadelphia: Lippincott.

Reynolds, S. (2000). The anatomy of evidence-based practice: Principles and methods. In L. Trinder & S. Reynolds (Eds.), *Evidence-Based Practice: A Critical Appraisal*. Malden, MA: Blackwell Science Ltd.

Roberts, A. R., & Yeager, K. (2004). Systematic reviews of evidence-based studies and practice-based research: How to search for, develop and use them. In A. R. Roberts & K. R. Yeager (Eds.), *Evidence-Based Practice Manual: Research and Outcome Measures in Health and Human Services*. Oxford, UK: University Press.

Sackett, D. L., Straus, S. E., Richardson, W. S., Rosenberg, W., & Haynes, R. B. (2000). *Evidence-Based Medicine: How to Practice & Teach EBM* (2nd ed.). London, UK: Churchill Livingstone.

Shorten, A., Wallace, M. C., & Crookes, P. A. (2001). Develop information literacy: A key to evidence-based nursing. *International Nursing Review, 48*(2), 86–92.

Stetler, C. B. (1994). Refinement of the Stetler/Marram model for application of research findings to practice. *Nursing Outlook, 42*(1), 15–25.

The Agency for Health Care Research and Quality Evidence-Based Practice Centers: Synthesizing scientific evidence to improve quality and effectiveness in healthcare. Available at: http://www.ahrg.gov/clinic/epc/. Accessed September 2, 2004.

Titler, M. G., Kleiber, C., Steelman, V. J., Rakel, B. A., Budreau, G., Everett, L. Q., Buckwalter, K. C., Tripp-Riemer, T., & Goode, C. J. (2001). The Iowa model of evidence-based practice to promote quality care. *Critical Care Nursing Clinics of North America, 13*(4), 497–509.

U.S. Department of Health and Human Services. (2000). The Registered Nurse Population March 2000: Findings from the National Sample Survey of Registered Nurses. Available at URL: http://bhpr.hrsa.gov/healthworkforce/reports/rnsurvey/rnss1.htm. Retrieved September 22, 2004.

Van Hoozer, H. L., Bratton, B. D., Ostmoe, P. M., Wienholtz, D., Craft, M. J., Albanese, M. A., & Gjerde, C. L. (1987). *The Teaching Process: Theory and Practice in Nursing*. Norwalk, CT: Appleton-Century-Crofts.

Wallace, M. C., Shorten, A., & Russell, K. G. (1997). Paving the way: Stepping stones to evidence-based nursing. *International Journal of Nursing Practice, 3*(3), 147–152.

Wallace, M. C., Shorten, A., Crookes, P. A., McGurk, C., & Brewer, C. (1999). Integrating information literacies into an undergraduate nursing programme. *Nurse Education Today, 19*(2), 136–141.

Wallace, M. C., Shorten, A., & Crookes, P. A. (2000). Teaching information literacy skills: An evaluation. *Nursing Education Today, 20*(6), 485–489.

Wheeler, K., Fasano, N., & Burr, L. (1995). Strategies for teaching research: A survey of baccalaureate programs. *Journal of Professional Nursing, 11*(4), 233–238.

CHAPTER 4

Linking Structure and Healing: Building Architecture for Evidence-Based Practice

Rosalyn Cama, FASID

The concept of designing buildings that engage our senses, envelope our psyche, and impact our well-being is nothing new. It is something we are subconsciously aware of, but rarely value.

Imagine planning an evening to celebrate one of those special life events. More than likely, you would search for a restaurant that offers excellent food, great ambiance, and superior service. You wouldn't select a restaurant that had not been renovated in 15 years, and had an unappealing view, vinyl tile floors, fluorescent lighting, loud ambient kitchen noise, and less-than-attentive wait staff who would ignore your table all evening. Even if the meal was great, would you consider that an appropriate setting for your special event?

Yet how many hospitals, where its visitors enter every day to experience special life-altering events, offer facilities much like the second restaurant described above? The available health services in that hospital may be extraordinary, but more than likely the facilities are substandard to our physical and psychological needs. Why then do we accept this kind of design for life-altering moments? As consumers, most of us are unaware of the statistics showing the impact that design has on our health outcome and—more importantly—on the performance of those who will serve us during our hospital stay. The onus is on those designing new facilities to consult proven evidence of factors that favorably impact behavioral, organizational, and economic outcomes.

This chapter addresses the link between structure and healing. It demonstrates how a process called evidence-based design (EBD) builds the strongest argument to design our healing facilities in an informed way. Let us first consider the historical links between structure and healing.

HISTORICAL PERSPECTIVE

> In a dark place the sick indulge themselves too much in various fancies, and are harassed by imaginings devised in an alienated mind, since no external phenomena can fall on the senses; but in a bright place they are prevented from being wholly in their own fancies, which are rather weakened by external phenomena.
> *Asclepiades of Bithynia, ca 50 bc* (Licht, 1955)

> Second only to fresh air...I should be inclined to rank light in importance for the sick. Direct sunlight, not only daylight, is necessary for speedy recovery. I mention from experience, as quite perceptible in promoting recovery, the being able to see out of a window, instead of looking against a dead wall; the bright colours of flowers; the being able to read in bed by the light of the window close to the bed-head. It is generally said the effect is upon the mind. Perhaps so, but it is not less so upon the body on that account.
> *Florence Nightingale, 1860* (Dover, 1969)

Obviously, the concept that our surroundings impact our well-being is not new. The recovery environment for patients, so succinctly described above, shows the importance of environmental attributes on patients' healing process. With such notable historical references to the healing environment, why has relatively little attention been given to this subject in contemporary design practices?

From a more modern perspective at how the economy has influenced the approach a professional designer takes to a health care project, hearken back to the recent past of the 1970s. During that period, the health care design specialty was known as "Institutional Design." The interior products available were nothing more than that, "institutional." Many were standard products from medical supply houses. During this same decade, much innovation was taking place in the corporate segment for the development of new building materials, interior finishes, textiles, and furnishings. The downturn in the economy in the early 1980s slowed production of those high-end products and sent a starving corporate sales force calling on the institutional design community. The beautiful finishes and expensive "bells and whistles" of the corporate product, however, were not acceptable to the emerging health care market. Designers turned to European suppliers, who were ahead of the American manufacturers, and they ordered many Scandinavian and German products from those who understood the ergonomic and maintenance issues of the health care environment. It was not long before U.S. office furniture makers retooled and stimulated competitiveness in the health care product industry.

Simultaneously, the whole economic structure of the health care industry changed. The cry from the newly formed Facilities Departments was to deliver a much more hospitable environment for patients who were turning into customers. It is said that it was the baby boomers, who were just starting their families, who demanded a new experience in birthing babies. Labor and Delivery Units across the country have not been the same since. Market pressure forced many hospitals to renovate and create a more home-like environment that encouraged participation from the father and extended family. As hospitals began to compete for this customer base, more market research was conducted. It was no surprise that support was found for this trend, which caused hospitable amenities to become standard hospital fare. The emergence at this very time of hospice was also no coincidence, as it too was driven by the same demographic needs of boomers preparing their parents for death and dying.

In 1988, a group of savvy professionals engaged in hospital consulting and design realized that the building and renovating of hospitals, primarily driven by the needs of medical practitioners and their new technologies, was missing an important participant in the final design solution. The patient and the host of caregivers, either clinical or family, were not being thoughtfully factored into the final design solutions. This band of innovators decided that those trying to take a broader approach to health care design should be highlighted in an annual conference. So was born the "Symposium on Healthcare Interior Design." This design conference focused on the areas of related research and aimed to educate a growing number of professionals already practicing in or entering this specialty. The originators of the Symposium have since created a more comprehensive learning experience and, in 2003, premiered "HEALTHCARE DESIGN." This annual conference draws in administrators, clinicians, practitioners and their project teams, and advocates who are making a difference in the way the patient and caregiver are accommodated in their hospital experience, to positively impact health, organizational, and economic outcomes.

The Center for Health Design, whose founders started the Symposium on Healthcare Design and produced it until 1998, was formed in 1993 as a research and advocacy organization. Through their research-based approach, The Center sought to find and sponsor some of the best research in the area of health care design. This effort continues to bring to light a host of emerging topics, as the health care industry continues to grow and become much more complex. The current mission of The Center for Health Design is to "transform healthcare settings into healing environments that improve outcomes through the creative use of evidence-based design" (2004, p. 1). To that end, The Center's vision is to, "Develop a future where healing environments are recognized as a vital part of therapeutic treatment, and where the design contributes to health and does not add to the burden of stress."

This nonprofit agency operates through the diligent efforts of a volunteer multidisciplinary board of directors and a committed host of dedicated committee members, who work toward a common goal of improving the settings in which health care is delivered. This group is comprised of researchers, architects, interior designers, health care chief executive officers (CEOs), physicians, nurse executives, quality improvement professionals, futurists, marketing, and fund-raising professionals. This is precisely the team make-up one would expect to find on a significant health care project's building team.

The nationwide list of new hospital building projects is remarkable. In the year 2004, there was approximately $17 billion of health care-related construction in the United States alone. The anticipated projection is for that number to grow to $25 billion by 2010.

"This is the strongest construction market in healthcare," said Robert Levine, Vice President of Turner Construction: Healthcare (Brandrud Company, 2003).

This increase in new building projects is attributed to the lack of capital investments in the most recent years; a shortage of hospital beds in most markets; bottlenecks in emergency departments, surgical suites, and intensive care units; and an increase in acuity levels as technology moves the less complicated case procedures into the out-patient arena. In addition, an aging population will tax this system as baby-boomers, already proven to instigate change in this and many other industries, enter an age of increased medical need. Taken together, these statistics are driving a stronger desire to have this discussion now and to build a body of knowledge that will help future projects.

Leland R. Kaiser, PhD, noted health care futurist, is attributed to having said, "The hospital is a human invention and can be reinvented at any time."

LOOKING TO THE PAST TO DETERMINE THE FUTURE

Three years after it began, The Center for Health Design engaged Haya Rubin, MD, PhD, to lead a team at Johns Hopkins University. Their task was to provide a literature search and analyze 30 years of research that had measured how the built environment and other environmental factors impacted patient health outcomes. Accepting only those studies with rigorous scientific methodologies, this Johns Hopkins-based team performed a meta-analysis of 78,761 publications, of which only 84 studies met their criteria.

Armed with this knowledge, the Center identified the following five areas that needed field study work (Center for Health Design, 1998):

1. Access to nature
2. Control of one's personal space
3. Positive distractions
4. Social support
5. Elimination of environmental stressors

The Center, along with Dr. Rubin's team, published these findings in the article, "Status Report: An Investigation to Determine Whether the Built Environment

Affects Patients' Health Outcomes," which is available on the Center's Web site (http://www.healthdesign.org).

The Center for Health Design next decided to explore consumer opinion to see where best to begin its research. In partnership with The Picker Institute (Cambridge, MA), patients and their families were asked two questions: what design strategies should be used to improve the quality of the physical environment and what matters in the environment.

This topic was not new to The Picker Institute. In the book, *Through the Patient's Eyes* (Gertis, Edgeman-Levitan, Daley, & Delbanco, 1993), the impact the design of a facility had on the perception of the quality of care already had been described. "By bringing the patient's perspective to the design and delivery of health services, providers can improve their ability to meet patients' needs and enhance the quality of care" (Center for Health Design & Picker Institute, 1997).

Nine two-hour focus groups were conducted that included three specific user groups: acute care, ambulatory care, and long-term care. The objective was to collect insights, attitudes, opinions, and perceptions from consumers about the physical environment of their hospital. The Center for Health Design and The Picker Institute recognized the need to capture the patient and family perspective, as defined by them as a means to:

> ....facilitate, integrate and accelerate the creation of life-enhancing environments. Patients and family members are increasingly being viewed as the experts in telling us what quality means to them—what matters, what makes them feel better and what things they need to support their recovery, healing and adaptation to significant life changes (Center for Health Design & Picker Institute, 1998).

Seven common themes emerged from this research. Consumers asked for a physical environment that:

1. Facilitates connection to staff
2. Is conducive to well-being
3. Is convenient and accessible
4. Is confidential and private
5. Is caring for the family
6. Is considerate of people's impairments
7. Is close to nature

Eight years later, the Robert Wood Johnson Foundation funded a project for the Center for Health Design to engage Roger Ulrich at Texas A&M and Craig Zimring at Georgia Tech to update the meta-analysis survey that had been done by Dr. Rubin and her team. This time, approximately 600 studies were discovered that met the standards for research rigor (Ulrich & Zimring, 2004). The intent of their project was to raise awareness in an industry that was investing a significant amount of money into capital improvements.

This updated survey found that the documented areas of evidence-based research primarily fell into three categories:

1. Environmental psychology, or how a building environment affects stress levels
2. Clinical research, or where the built environment impacts the medical and scientific approach to care
3. Administrative studies, or how the built environment affects the management of their institution

A small body of research in the areas of evolutionary biology and neuroscience was also discovered.

In the environmental psychology studies, they found outcomes related to areas where social support was needed to promote health and healing. The degree of control persons had over their environment not only impacted their own health outcomes, but also performance issues related to their caregivers. Positive distractions were found to be a factor that eliminated stress. Countless studies showed a direct correlation between the impact nature and health outcomes, particularly when considering the length of stay. Ulrich's landmark 1984 study set the standard for what a patient views from his or her bed; those patients who had a view of nature versus a brick wall had a shorter length of hospital stay (Ulrich, 2004).

WHAT IS EVIDENCE-BASED DESIGN?

EBD is the deliberate attempt to base building design decisions on the best available evidence. In a survey of the Center for Health Design's board, the factors most likely to influence building design relate specifically to:

1. Patient outcomes
2. Staff recruitment and retention
3. Quality of service
4. Improved medical safety procedures
5. Operational efficiency
6. Financial performance

Rationale for Evidence-Based Design

We know that a visit to a health care facility is one of the most stressful events in a person's life. People often enter a facility anxious about the treatment or illness. Add pain to the mix and the odds for increased stress go up. Now, with that condition in mind, most hospitals offer a self-serve model to negotiate the halls of their facilities, one of the most complex forms of architecture in terms of way-finding. Once admitted, the current model in health care is to withhold most information and parse out only what the patient needs to know, thus taking away personal control. Add one caregiver who is overworked and needs an attitude adjustment, and you have a perfect recipe for overwhelming frustration and stress. Most likely he or she has issues outside of the hospital-related stress that compound the situation. That cranky caregiver may be in conflict with a colleague or other family member; he or she may be facing an unrealistic workload; or the fears about his or her seriously ill loved one may be overwhelming. These and a myriad of other factors add to the recipe for stress.

For both patient and relatives, these factors psychologically engender a sense of helplessness, anxiety, and/or depression. Physiologically, blood pressure increases, and there are increased muscle tension and higher levels of circulating stress hormones. Behaviorally, a patient may respond with a verbal outburst, social withdrawal, passivity, sleeplessness, alcohol or other drug abuse, and/or noncompliance with medication orders.

Few studies have examined health care workplace performance, but much can be learned by following the research done in other design industries. In 1998, the American Society of Interior Designers (ASID) conducted a study entitled, "Workplace Performance," to explore how design can influence performance and change corporate culture. It led to a deeper understanding of how interior surroundings can contribute to an improved work life. Although it was conducted in corporate environments, this study identified five key components to creating a productive workplace:

1. People performance
2. Designed environment
3. Workflow
4. Technology
5. Human resources

When the designed environment was explored further, four design factors were noted to improve productivity (American Society of Interior Designers, 1998):

1. Access to people and resources
2. Comfort in one's surroundings
3. Privacy
4. Flexibility of the environment

These four design factors not only contribute to how to improve staff productivity, but also how to enhance recruitment and retention efforts. In a subsequent ASID study entitled, "Retaining and Recruiting Employees through

Design," it was found that following compensation, design of the work environment was tied for second with benefits when ranking an employee's decision to accept or stay with a job. In both of these studies, the built environment is known to influence productivity and reduce work force turnover (ASID, 1998).

These early qualitative studies that the Center for Health Design and ASID conducted in the late 1990s mark a flashpoint in the thinking about how design is perceived to influence human behavior, and the need to educate a design profession about how current research can inform their design solutions. One outcome was that the ASID, in a joint venture with the University of Minnesota, created a Web-based clearinghouse for all research being conducted in all design specialties. The result of this effort is the Web site named "Informedesign" (http://www.informedesign). Intended to be a communications tool, it is updated on a weekly basis. Its hope is to make the effort of finding research to support design issues as easy as searching for a product. It is a start to make a behavioral change in the design process.

At the same time, The American Institute of Architects together with the American Academy of Neuroscience for Architecture formed an effort to study how the brain responds to the built environment. Their goal was to determine how it may be possible through the application of neuroscience research to understand the impact of architectural settings on human emotions, moods, and behaviors. This effort marked an important collaborative step with multiple specialties to focus on the impact the built environment has on human behavior. (More information can be found at: http://www.aia.org.)

In a follow-up to the Robert Wood Johnson Foundation research, a conference was convened in June 2004 that spoke directly to the transformation needed in the hospital work environment. Using a holistic approach that addresses the "mind, body, and spirit" of hospitals, Project Leader Victoria Weisfeld made the connection clearly. The "mind" part of the equation refers to work design and process in hospitals; the "body" focuses on the physical design of the hospital workplace; and the "spirit" refers to the soul of an organization, which is its vitality, values, attitudes, or simply put, its culture (Weisfeld, 2004).

THE REVOLUTIONARY PEBBLE PROJECT

The Center for Health Design found that the next step in approaching this important design issue was to develop a multi-year field research project. Field research has been difficult because of the number of variables that can influence an outcome. Working with a group of academic researchers, the Center devised a way to overcome most of these variables.

"The Pebble Project," as this amazing research project is known, aims to work with progressive health care organizations throughout the world that are engaged in significant building projects, and believe in the potentially beneficial relationship between the facility design process, the ultimate facility design, and organizational behavior. The Center for Health Design believes that, just as a pebble tossed into a pond creates a ripple effect, well-researched and documented examples of projects demonstrating the benefit of these relationships will ripple through the health care and design communities.

There are two unique components of this Pebble Project. The first is its emphasis on understanding how organizational behavior changes because of the planning and design process. The second is the development of a standardized evaluation methodology that in turn leads to:

- Comparison of outcomes
- Identification of best practices
- Continuous improvements of health care design

Timing Is Everything

When a number of people begin to feel the same pain about a topic at the same time, usually a movement begins. As we can see, a convergence of thinking was going on in the late 1990s. In 1998, The Institute of Medicine (IOM) issued a "Statement on Quality of Care" for our health care system. IOM described quality care as care that is patient-centered, efficient, effective, safe, equitable, and timely. Although the thinking was about how a system of health delivery could improve its culture and, hence, behavior, the Center for Health Design examined this mantra in an effort to understand how the built environment can support such behavioral changes. The questions raised helped to form the research matrix of the Pebble Project (Table 4.1). The results currently being gathered in the Pebble Project are supporting the Center's initial hypotheses.

This research matrix is being used to advise hospitals on research possibilities. It is also used by the Center for Health Design to determine when multiple hospitals are reporting on the same hypotheses.

The IOM's Statement on Quality of Care correlation to the Pebble Project's initial results is simply described below.

Patient-Centered

In a customer-driven society, why would we even consider less than a private room? Costs to deliver care, you say? Well, do we really know the effect that the sharing of a space has on a health outcome, on the effectiveness of family-provided care, or on the flexibility a room designed for variable acuity can have on operational costs? If you provide positive distractions, will the experience be less stress-

Table 4.1   Pebble Project Research Matrix

Comparative Group → Outcome Research ↓	Patients (S, G, or A)	Employees/ Physicians (S, G, or A)	Family/Visitors (S, G, A)	Community	Organization/ Institution
Clinical/Technical Outcomes		N/A	N/A	N/A	N/A
Economic/Financial Resource Utilization					
Operational Improvements				N/A	
Satisfaction, Quality of Life, Cultural Assessment					
Safety/Error Reduction Outcomes			N/A		N/A
Environmental/ Sustainability					
Other Measurable Outcomes					

Project Name: _____

Explanation of S, G, or A:
Research studies can be designed to look at the effects as follows:

1. **S = Same** (identical) group of patients, families, or employees pre- and post-intervention.
   a. Sickle cell patients admitted to an old unit vs. the same patients admitted to a new unit
   b. Patients undergoing knee replacement of one knee in old unit vs. other knee in new unit
   c. Same mothers giving birth in old unit vs. new unit

2. **G = Group** (type/group) of patients, families, or employees pre- and post-intervention.
   a. Patients of a particular diagnostic type
   b. Patients treated in a particular unit or in a particular office
   c. Employees in a particular work group
   d. Families of hospitalized children

3. **A = All** (the entire population) of patients, families, or employees pre- and post-intervention.

ful? If access to information using resource libraries or computer terminals answers more questions, will the patient feel a partnership in his or her care? To date, the Pebble Project research has yielded great support for a patient-centered approach. With four Pebble Projects reporting on collected data, the following was noted:

(Saint Alphonsus Regional Medical Center, Boise, ID)
"Noise levels have been reduced by designing larger private rooms, adding carpet

to the hallways, putting acoustical tiles on the walls and ceilings, and relocating machinery and nurse charting away from patients."
"Average decibel rate per patient room was less than 51.7."
"Quality of sleep improved 4.9 to 7.3 (on a scale of 0–10)."
"Patient satisfaction scores improved during a three-month comparison period."

(Bronson Methodist Hospital, Kalamazoo, MI)
"Private patient rooms have resulted in decreased patient transfers because of the elimination of conflicts among patients that necessitated moves and an increase in patient sleep quality."
"Built environment survey found that private rooms made for a better patient experience and that it enables higher quality of patient care."

Timely

In any service-based business, timing is everything. The questions are: How can we deliver quality care in an environment that supports redundancy of motion, which does not support increased access to patients, or improve communications between staff and patients and their family members? By understanding the tasks at hand to deliver care, studying the time and motion required to deliver that care, challenging conventional delivery models, and improving visual and physical access, the quality of care improves. The amount of bedside care delivered increases, hence, improving staff satisfaction among nurses, since this is why they went into nursing in the first place. The net result is a reduction in turnover rates.

Technology has increased the patient's access to medical knowledge at home, so why restrict that flow of information in a health setting? Communications can be timely, not only delivered at the bedside, but also in community conference centers, patient- and family-accessible resource libraries, and Internet accessible dataports to a hospital Web-based information center located in waiting rooms. As more hospitals offer private rooms, waiting rooms become obsolete, and these are perfect locations to create patient floor resource centers.

Evidence from Pebble Research includes the following:

(Bronson Methodist Hospital, Kalamazoo, MI)
"Overall satisfaction increased to 95.4%"
"Nursing turnover rates are below 12%"
"Market share has increased 6%"
"Employee satisfaction has improved"

(Methodist Hospital/Clarian Health Partners, Indianapolis, IN)
"Overall patient dissatisfaction dropped from 6% in 1998 to 3% in 2001."

(The Barbara Ann Karmanos Cancer Institute, Detroit, MI)
"Patient satisfaction rose 18%."
"Nurse attrition fell from 23% to 3.8%."

Efficiency

When dealing with the health of humankind, why would we, as a society, expect less than efficient work processes in the setting that delivers our care? Yet most facilities are antiquated and ridden with processes that were the best in their day, but need serious redefinition given today's technology. Do patients need to be transferred to services that are now mobile?

Pebble Research is showing:

(Methodist Hospital/Clarian Health Partners, Indianapolis, IN)
"Patient room layout, equipment integration, and other design features have helped push patient transfers down 90%."

(Methodist Hospital/Clarian Health Partners, Indianapolis, IN)
"Caregiver workload index has been reduced, resulting in improvements in nursing efficiency."

(The Barbara Ann Karmanos Cancer Institute, Detroit, MI)
"Lower daily variable costs per case."

Equitable

Is health care different for the "haves" and the "have-nots"? We all know that should not be true, but a recent Yale University study found that African Americans and Hispanics suffering severe heart attacks must wait significantly longer than whites for emergency treatment at hospitals. The delays are largely due to the poor quality of the hospitals that minorities typically use. These hospitals (that serve these populations) may lack up-to-date communications and diagnostic equipment and could be poorly organized (Bradley et al., 2004).

Efficacy

If the goal of medicine is "to do no harm," then in addition to their role of the caregiver, what responsibilities do the facility managers have in that statement? We know that the amount of disruption in an environment and the quality of sleep have direct effects on healing. We know that private rooms, the location of sinks, and the rate of air exchange decreases infection rates. Elimination of environmental stressors such as noise, glare, odor, and poor air quality, and the addition of adequate way-finding also lower stress.

Pebble Research shows, with improved design:

(The Barbara Ann Karmanos Cancer Institute, Detroit, MI)
"Reduced pain medication requirements and decreased medication variances."

Safety

It is normal to expect that a facility that is designed to deliver the care for your health is also a safe environment, but that is not always so. Obstacles contribute to patient falls; medical orders are misunderstood because of acoustical distractions; there is a lack of physical organization; storage for just-in-time material delivery reduces efficiency in the delivery of care; and lack of proper hand-washing or air exchange rates increases the risk of hospital-borne (nosocomial) infections.

Pebble Research evidence found:

(Bronson Methodist Hospital, Kalamazoo, MI)
"Private rooms, location of sinks and airflow design have resulted in an 11% overall decrease in nosocomial infections."

(Methodist Hospital/Clarian Health Partners, Indianapolis, IN)
"Patient falls are down 75% due to the unit's decentralized design, which allows for better observation."
"Decrease in patient transfers and nurses' more consistent knowledge of each patient's condition has contributed to an improved medication error index."

(The Barbara Ann Karmanos Cancer Institute, Detroit, MI)
"30% reduction in medical errors, a result of increased space in medication room, location of medication room, organization of medical supplies, standardized visual cues, and acoustical panels to decrease noise levels."
"6% reduction in patient falls, a result of better visualization of patients due to angle of doorway, improved lighting, and room layout."

A GROWING BODY OF EVIDENCE

Timing is everything. When a group of innovators presents a strong enough case to push a new concept, others will follow as soon as the risk level is diminished. The above-noted research that the built environment does in fact impact behavior is no longer a hypothesis. In the health care segment of design, we now have the Pebble Project's ongoing work to build the case for unrefutable proof. As more and more hospitals add to that body of knowledge, we will see what futurist Daniel Burrus (1993) refers to as a "flashpoint," and what is now seen as a solution to spend discretionary dollars may, in fact, become code. It is this transformation in thinking that is the hope of those who have learned to rely on an evidence-based approach to hypothesize, measure, and then design solutions.

In their literature search, Drs. Ulrich and Zimring (2004) found four basic assumptions where there is a compelling amount of research to drive design decisions:

1. By reducing staff stress/fatigue, the effectiveness in delivering care increases.
2. By changing design, patient safety and quality of care improve.
3. By reducing patient stress, the quality of life and healing for patients and families improves.
4. By improving overall health quality, costs will be reduced.

In their first assumption, "by reducing staff stress/fatigue the effectiveness in delivering care increases," these authors found overwhelming evidence that reducing noise levels in the work environment and improving job satisfaction will create positive outcomes. To a lesser degree, improving medication processing and delivery times, improving work effectiveness, and increasing patient care time per shift achieve the same outcome. Other studies show a correlation between improving the workplace and job satisfaction, reduced fatigue, and reduction in turnover rates.

Their second assumption, "by changing design, patient safety and quality of care improve," without a doubt, is achieved by reducing the rates of airborne and contact nosocomial infections. Improving communication between all parties involved in care, reducing the number of patient falls and medication errors, improving confidentiality of patient information, and increasing hand-washing compliance by staff all have proven positive outcomes.

In their third assumption, "by reducing patient stress, the quality of life and healing for patients and families improves," there is a tremendous amount of work showing a direct correlation when noise is reduced, spatial disorientation is minimized, sleep quality improves, and social support increases, which reduces patient stress (emotional, duress, anxiety, and depression). Fewer studies are offered suggesting that reducing depression, improving circadian rhythms, reducing feelings of helplessness, and empowering patients and families, providing positive distractions, and reducing pain (intake of pain drugs and reported pain) affect outcomes.

In their final assumption, "by improving overall health quality, costs will be reduced," it is without doubt that the reduction of patient transfers and improving quality of care offer the best results. To a lesser degree, patient outcomes are affected by staff work effectiveness or increased patient care time per shift, reduction in the length of stay, reduction in the administration of drugs, patient satisfaction as it relates to staff quality, and finally, re-hospitalization or re-admission rates (Center for Health Design, 2004).

The beauty of this report is that it helps quantify where much work has already been done. These studies give us the clues as to where to form our design hypotheses for design solutions. Although a prescriptive solution is not so easy, the Pebble Project provides us with a framework to begin to understand how best to create structured, individual research projects that can achieve the right solutions in each of these areas for a given design problem. The Center for Health Design also offers guidance in this process.

A TRADITION BASED ON TRUST

Like so many better ideas and products, if they come to market before their time, then their impact is lost on a society that is just not ready. Results gained from these early research projects must now be introduced into practice to inform upcoming design decisions. This process—an evidence-based approach—is not new to the design field; it is just uncommon outside of the ivy halls of academia. Much research has already proven that the built environment does have an impact on human behavior. The problem, however, is that design professionals (including architects, interior designers, landscape architects, graphic designers, etc.) have relied mostly on an interview process, time-honored design principles, and experience to justify solutions. Over time, building codes and regulatory guidelines have ensured that the most obvious and sometimes proven solutions that pertain to health, safety, and welfare have been applied. Within the confines of a building project, it is rare that the processes of hypothesis, measurement, and outcome determination are integrated and supportive of an evidence-based approach. It is ironic that in the health care field, where medical practice is built on measurement and improving outcomes, the same does not hold true for its design consultants.

In an August 2000 *Lancet* article, Colin Martin wrote, "Although the premise that the physical environment affects well-being reflects common sense, evidence-based design is poised to emulate evidence-based medicine as a central tenet for healthcare in the 21st century" (Martin, 2000).

Selection Process of Qualified Design Consultants

Most design consultants come to their client's table by presenting the best examples of their previous projects. A portfolio of similar projects, an understanding of the client's goals, their design process, decision-making skills, ability to build consensus, ability to manage both budgets and schedule, and team compatibility are often the qualifiers for project awards. This is a blatant example of a "trust me" model. This approach does not fail, but it is devoid of measurement with quantifiable results, thus proving the building's impact on health outcomes and workplace performance. This is just a shift in qualifying a consultant with measurable outcomes or EBD.

A good practitioner is trained in interviewing skills and will take a soft approach to the more rigorous scientific model to measure, draw conclusions, and develop intuitive hypotheses that will prove that a proposed solution is sound. Is this wrong? Many great buildings and memorable interiors have been built in this less than scientific way, but many great opportunities in design also have been missed because of a misunderstanding of a design feature's impact on the behavior of the building's occupants. The real sacrifice is made when a project's budget needs to be shaved—a process we irreverently call "value-engineering," where decisions are made to arbitrarily remove a value-added feature with no justification other than to cut the project's capital expenditure. Since very little evidence exists to correlate the design's operational impact, the feature is deleted.

If we could expect a "show me" model to the design process, then decision-making would refer to past evidence in similar scenarios to help hypothesize a new scenario. This new scenario would have to be tested again to reveal if it proved worthy in the new situation. When enough data are gathered to support a supposition, the design feature should inform a new code or design guideline. With the number of building projects that occur on an annual basis, it would not be long before a substantial body of knowledge would inform a more evidence-based approach to project decisions. The caution is that these individual research projects not lead to "cookie cutter" solutions. The intent—and this is an important point—is that the process should lead to an evolutionary way to improve the design of our health care facilities. As there are ever-changing advances in medical care, technology, and societal needs, so shall our design solutions evolve and not remain stagnant.

In a November 2003 "Healthcare Design" article, "The Four Levels of Evidence-Based Practice," D. Kirk Hamilton best described the roles of design consultants. Hamilton defined the practitioner's tasks as follows (Hamilton, 2003, p. 18):

- Study the available research and interpretation of the implications for design
- Hypothesize the intended results of a design intervention and measure the outcomes

- Share the results publicly to advance the field
- Subject the results to peer review and the validity of academic rigor

Table 4.2 expands on these "Four Levels" by outlining a few practical ways that designers can achieve a better practice.

Table 4.2   Four Stages of Evidence-Based Practice

	Activity	Level 1	Level 2	Level 3	Level 4
Interpret the Evidence	Read material to stay current on emerging research	★	★	★	★
	Use critical thinking to interpret implications of research on current projects	★	★	★	★
	Collect success stories and historical data on completed projects	★	★	★	★
Hypothesize & Measure	Perform applied research as a practitioner on real projects		★	★	★
	Hypothesize intended results of design interventions		★	★	★
	Measure the results associated with design interventions		★	★	★
Share Results Publicly	Report unbiased project results in the public arena, writing and speaking			★	★
	Perform independent 3rd party post-occupancy evaluations			★	★
	Obtain advanced educations to improve understanding of research methods			★	★
Meet Academic Standards	Collaborate with credible academic researchers and social scientists				★
	Publish research results in peer-reviewed journals				★
	Complete academic thesis or dissertation on evidence-based design topic				★

Source: HEALTHCARE DESIGN Magazine, 2003. Reprinted with the permission of D. Kirk Hamilton.

A PROCESS DEFINED

The process of planning, programming, designing, and building a new facility is well established and proven to deliver award-winning results. The idea of taking an evidence-based approach is not intended to challenge that methodology, but is only to enhance it. The best way to begin a project is with a clear expectation of what is to be accomplished in the effort of building a new facility or renovating the existing facility. It is here that the partnership between consultant and client needs to be strong. Time and time again it has been shown that what makes a project great is that it is client-driven by a strong vision. This vision is not just an inspiring phrase crafted during an administrative retreat. It must be an image emotionally owned by all who are involved in a building project for what is being created for an institution's future. It is that insight that will make a consultant's role in hypothesizing design and, hence, behavioral outcomes more realistic. The financial investment when measured and evaluated will be justifiably clear.

In his book, *Discovering the Soul of Service*, Berry (1999) identifies the nine drivers of successful leadership as follows:

1. Value-driven leadership
2. Strategic focus
3. Executional excellence
4. Control of destiny
5. Trust-based relationships
6. Investment in employee success
7. Acting small
8. Brand cultivation
9. Company's generosity

Berry's ingredients for such leadership will empower a design team (outside consultants as well as internal committees) to produce their best work. Add to this mix a willingness and ability to reference the literature searches for proven outcomes, develop a hypothesis for the project's outcome, and then measure unique differences in the subject's environment. It is then that the conventional design process can be transformed so that a noteworthy project can be built where behaviors will be changed with clear and full understanding of the intended outcomes.

FUTURE EXPECTATIONS ARE FOREVER CHANGED

In 2004, Leonard L. Berry, Derek Parker, Russell C. Coile, Jr., D. Kirk Hamilton, David D. O'Neill, and Blair L. Sadler (all current or past board members of the

Center for Health Design) developed a futurist's perspective of a hospital and how it could function after applying the known principles learned from The Pebble Research Project. This compilation of known outcomes was written as a fictitious parable entitled, the "Fable Hospital." Fable was defined as a form of imaginative literature constructed in such a way that readers are encouraged to look for meanings hidden beneath the literal surface of the fiction (Berry et al., 2004).

These authors describe this hospital as a 300-bed regional medical center built to replace a 50-year-old facility that had 250 beds. Located on an urban site, the facility provides a comprehensive range of inpatient and ambulatory services with a cost for replacement of $240 million. The assumption is made that leadership and operational core values are outstanding and clearly administered, that the design protocol is truly evidence-based, and that research is ongoing throughout the design process.

Added features include what is now proven, including oversized rooms maximizing outdoor views and daylight exposure; acuity adaptable rooms with state-of-the-art monitoring and communications technology; double door bathroom access; decentralized barrier-free nursing; alcohol-rub hand hygiene dispensers as needed; HEPA filtration; built-in flexibility for future technology growth; peaceful settings creating necessary distractions; noise reducing measures; private consultation areas; patient education centers on each floor; and staff support facilities that reduce stress. These design upgrades cost the project an additional $12 million. In a CEO report to the hospital board, after the first year of operation where outcomes were carefully measured, the incremental costs are virtually recovered after one year and significant financial benefit will accrue year after year.

Although this is all a supposition, it is backed by ongoing research in an ever-growing area. The report fully describes the cost expenditures and savings, and is worth studying if you are to engage in a building project. This database of knowledge will grow as this movement continues.

JOIN A MOVEMENT THAT IS PROVEN

This chapter only begins to link structure and healing. It is an exciting new field that is getting the attention it deserves. If you are engaged in designing or building, then it is important to fully understand the evidence-based approach to design, embrace it, and invest in the methodology before you begin your next building project. This body of knowledge is changing daily and can change a life-altering health-related event that we will all experience personally or through a loved one at some time during our lives.

Close your eyes and imagine the place where you like to escape to after a stressful period. Focus on the elements of that environment that support your sense of well-being. Design your hospital of the future with those qualities in mind, using the known evidence to justify their expenditures and not value-engineer out those factors that make us heal.

REFERENCES

American Society of Interior Designers. (1998). *Productive Workplaces: How Design Increases Productivity: Expert Insights.* Washington, DC: ASID.

Asclepiades. (1955). *Asclepiades, his life and writings.* New Haven, CT: Licht Publishing.

Berry, L. (1999). *Discovering the Soul of Service: Nine Drivers of Sustainable Business Success.*

Berry, L., Parker, D., Coile, R., Hamilton, K., O'Neill, D., & Sadler, B. (2004). *Can Better Buildings Improve Care and Increase Your Financial Returns?* Chicago, IL: ACHE/HAP.

Bradley, E. H., Herrin, J., Wang, Y., McNamara, R. I., Webster, T. R., et al. (2004). Racial and ethnic differences in time to acute reperfusion therapy for patients hospitalized with myocardial infarction. *JAMA, 292*(13), 1563–1572.

Transforming Medical Institutions into Cultures of Caring. Brandrud company brochure. (2003).

Burrus, D. (1993). *Technotrends: How to Use Technology to Go Beyond Your Competition,* New York: Harper Business.

Center for Health Design. (2004). *Preliminary Report for Designing the 21st Century Hospital Symposium.* Washington, DC: Center for Health Design.

Center for Health Design. (1998). *Status Report: An Investigation to Determine Whether the Built Environment Affects Patients' Medical Outcomes.* Martinez.

Center for Health Design & The Picker Institute. (1997). *Consumer Perceptions of the Healthcare Environment: An Investigation to Determine What Matters.* Martinez.

"Designing the 21st Century Hospital" conference. Sponsored by the Robert Wood Johnson Foundation and the Center for Health Design, Washington, DC, June, 2004.

Gerteis, M., Edgeman-Levitan, S., Daley, J., & Delbanco, T. L. (1993). *Through the Patient's Eyes: Understanding and Promoting Patient Centered Care.* San Francisco: Jossey-Bass.

Hamilton, K. (2003). *The Four Levels of Evidence-Based Practice.* Washington, DC: HEALTHCARE DESIGN, pp. 18–26.

Martin, C. (2000). Transported by the architecture of London's new Underground. *LANCET.* 356(9233); 947–948.

Nightingale, F. (1969). *Notes on Nursing: What it is and what it is not.* Mineola, NY: Dover Publications.

Symposium on Healthcare Design. Sponsored by Imark Communications and The Center for Health Design, Anaheim, CA, 2000.

Ulrich, R., & Zimring, C. (2004). *The Role of the Physical Environment in the Hospital of the 21st Century: A Once in a Lifetime Opportunity.* Concord, CA: The Center for Health Design.

CHAPTER 5

Living Evidence:
Translating Research into Practice

Marie P. Farrell

THE CALF-PATH

One day, through the primeval wood,
A calf walked home, as good calves should;
But made a trail all bent askew,
A crooked trail, as all calves do.

Since then three hundred years have fled,
And, I infer, the calf is dead.
But still he left behind his trail,
And thereby hangs my moral tale.

* * *

The years passed on in swiftness fleet.
The road became a village street,
And this, before men were aware,
A city's crowded thoroughfare,
And soon the central street was this
Of a renowned metropolis;
And men two centuries and a half
Trod in the footsteps of that calf.

Each day a hundred thousand rout
Followed that zigzag calf about,
And o'er his crooked journey went
The traffic of a continent.
A hundred thousand men were led
By one calf near three centuries dead.

They follow still his crooked way,
And lose one hundred years a day,
For thus such reverence is lent
To well-established precedent.

A moral lesson this might teach,
Were I ordained and called to preach;
For men are prone to go it blind
Along the calf-paths of the mind,
And work away from sun to sun
To do what other men have done.
They follow in the beaten track,
And out and in, and forth and back,
And still their devious course pursue,
To keep the path that others do.

They keep the path a sacred groove,
Along which all their lives they move,
But how the wise old wood-gods laugh,
Who saw the first primeval calf!
Ah! Many things this tale might teach—
But I am not ordained to preach.

Sam Walter Foss (1858–1911)

Ancient chronicles tell how, for a thousand years, the Kazakhstan city of Alma-Ata gave a friendly welcome to the trade caravans that journeyed along the Great Silk Road between Europe and the Far East. For centuries, traders followed the old familiar path to Alma Ata until the discovery of new sea routes. Then the old path was gradually abandoned. It was in this city of this most ancient of trade routes that in 1978, the World Health Organization (WHO) held its summit on the future of global health care. Financial experts, governmental officials, attorneys, health officials, nurses, physicians, and other health providers from over 168 countries gathered to map out new paths for health care into the next century.

The result of their efforts was a call for perhaps the most revolutionary health care reforms ever made: The Alma Ata Declaration and Health for All by the Year 2000 (HFA 2000). Health care, the delegates declared, had to be universally accessible to individuals and families in the community by means acceptable to them, through their full participation, and at a cost the individual, community, and country could afford (Primary Health Care, 1978, p. 34). This declaration became the cornerstone of the WHO regional and worldwide efforts to think globally and act locally.

The local version of the declaration in the United States was Healthy People 2000 and, more recently, Healthy People 2010. The European regional version was the Thirty-Eight Regional Targets for Health. Regardless of region, however, the approach to health was to be through primary health care (PHC). Nursing was to play a major role in PHC, to continue to map its path from the time of Florence Nightingale, through the years of the Alma Ata Declaration, through a century of practice and research to the present—a time some characterize as a chaotic period in health care.

This chapter examines the ways in which nursing has evolved within the context of a tumultuous period of events, both within and outside of the health care industry, and how it has distinguished itself from "doing what other men have done" by carving out its unique contribution through a series of developmental steps. One of these, the subject of this chapter, is the translation of research into evidence-based practice, a step that has brought both opportunities and challenges to the discipline as well as to the patients and communities that require nursing services.

IMPLICATIONS OF ALMA ATA

The implications of the Alma Ata Declaration on the delivery of nursing and the evolution to evidence-based practice are considerable. Major shifts in thinking had to occur because millions of people throughout the world had little or no access to care despite the burgeoning health-related industries in many countries (Parker, 2002). The intent was to ensure quality care and to place the individual at the center, to have access to knowledge, information, and resources for treating diseases and maintaining high levels of wellness, for a life span that might extend into one's nineties. This was to be accomplished in ways that would be appropriate, culturally acceptable, and affordable.

This affordable health care was to shift from the top down, from large bureaucratic institutions to locally managed health services. Governments, at the time, struggled with the burgeoning costs of their health services, owed in part to the advances underway in computer technology, genetic engineering, organizational development, communication technology, and thinking about ways to work smarter at a lower cost. As the health community worked to integrate the explosion of knowledge and technology, a similar pattern of change was underway in Asia in a field unrelated to health care.

The 1980s

A worldwide transformation occurred after World War II, when Deming (2000) traveled to Japan to help rebuild the country. This initiative launched the total quality movement that emerged into the drive for continuous quality improvement (CQI). (The name most associated with quality, however, was Donabedian [1980, 1988], who emphasized the key elements of structure, process, and outcome, the traces of which can be found in today's literature on evidence-based practice.)

Throughout the 1980s, WHO promoted HFA 2000, Europe, its Thirty-Eight Regional Targets for Health (Targets for HFA, 1991), and the United States, its Healthy People 2000. These initiatives, in part, helped to focus attention on a concrete, albeit medically oriented set of health care outcomes. The inspired initiatives of WHO also emphasized an inductive process from the individual client to the office of the caretaker, to the community, to regional, national, and international levels of health care. PHC providers developed the PHC system to support their services. Now they would use the same system to process their surrogate measure of success: data.

Data as Evidence

Data would be key to this process, along with its measurement and its generalizability. As Pirsig observed in his cavalier analysis of the metaphysics of quality, "Data without generalization is just gossip" (1991, p. 5). Clearly, the importance of data as evidence, its measurement, and its application would be critical, as would its generalized use beyond the immediate research setting. However, effective measurement would, in turn, depend on the knowledge of what should be measured, and this knowledge would be generated from the bottom up. Data would be used to compare best practices and to support innovation across hospital units, cities, regions, and countries. With increasing sophistication, countries could compare the relative number, type, and intensity or "dose" of interventions carried out as well as their costs, and ultimately, the funding of practices that met the test of being based, not on intuition, but on evidence. In this regard, the very essence of practice became an issue of concern at the governmental level, and the business of funding evidence-based practices would emerge as a transformative force to promote these practices, as financial transactions to benefit from them, or, as some fear, to control them (Winch, Creedy, & Chaboyer, 2002).

Research, Evidence, and Costs

One of evidence-based practice's precursors, then, was the quality movement. After Japan, it appeared in the United States at Florida Power and Light and found leadership in Dr. Brent James at Intermountain Health Care in Utah. Gradually, total quality management (TQM) was replaced by total quality improvement, and still later by CQI. Dr. Don Berwick in Massachusetts, among others, demonstrated unique approaches to data, their quality, and their measurement. Deming, Juran, and others who wrote during this period insisted that management was responsible for outcomes and had to take a leadership role to ensure these outcomes throughout the health care system (Juran, 1989, Juran 1992).

The effects of this movement were widespread. The insurance industry saw reduced premium payouts and approaches to lowering the enormous health care costs that put some companies out of business. Administrators in the health care industry found a reduction in lawsuits as concrete steps could be identified from the beginning of a visit to the health care provider, through the system, and either an exit from the system or an internal next step to treatment, care, and rehabilitation, all in a prearranged, timely manner understood by those involved. The European Union established funding sources for projects in this area and worked to "normalize" practices across the region. Canada and Australia made similar changes, and government agencies came to recognize nursing as a major force in the quality initiative.

Europeans undertook the most extensive study of nursing care ever funded at national levels in Europe during the 1980s (Farrell, 1987a, 1987b), and the National Institute of Nursing Research, under Hinshaw's leadership, launched and maintained nursing's national research agenda consistent with that of the nation's health agenda. Funded studies focused on the practice of nursing that, again, met the criteria of PHC and encouraged the further specification of practices in which nurses engaged that would yield the greatest results at costs that were affordable.

Organizations, including health care organizations, throughout the country created quality teams, and hospitals held hours of meetings during which health care providers were trained as leaders and facilitators. Tired pediatricians, unit secretaries, nursing's clinical specialists, group leaders, and facilitators sat discussing the flow-through of a piece of equipment from the loading dock to the patient's bedside, all in the name of horizontal processing, to ensure the right equipment, at the right bedside, for the right patient, under the right conditions. Quality teams described these efforts in words not unlike the PHC philosophy about care, provided in a manner that was appropriate, and delivered in a manner that was, again, culturally appropriate, acceptable, and cost effective.

Soon, however, hospitals found that the discipline-packed teams got weary of endless meetings that met over extended periods. Team work activities took precious time from other duties and, most importantly, the crucial element in practice was *not* time-on-task, but the best practice that resulted and could be compared to others' results through a comparative analysis called benchmarking.

Comparing Evidence

While hospitals and health services were comparing best practices, patients were comparing worst practices, and became vocal and persistent in the process. As the acquired immune deficiency syndrome (AIDS) epidemic galloped through the eighties and into the nineties, bright, articulate, young people with human immunodeficiency virus (HIV) insisted on being involved in their care and, in part, contributed to the sweeping changes among consumers (Shilts, 1987). The Internet emerged with a consumer movement that was to change the way all were to view health and its ownership. Government, insurers, the hospitals, health care providers, and the consumer were moving toward ways of knowing unprecedented in health care's history.

In industry, just-in-time philosophies invaded manufacturing and other organizations that sold products (Goldratt & Fox, 1986). Just how many greeting cards did Hallmark have to keep ready in its storehouse, anyway? And who were the people who really made a difference to a company? Did a bank really need all those tellers? Why not improve the way banking services were delivered, and at the same time, so went the argument, reduce costs by placing workers in part-time positions, thereby reducing, or eliminating altogether, their health care coverage?

Health care was now at a premium, and only those practices that could result in data that evidenced concrete change would be referred, counted, and paid for. Further, this evidence was to be located at the site of the interface between the customer (read patient) and the organization (read nurse).

This locus of control was shifting from the traditional banking teller and customer to a wall of a bank building with an ATM machine attached, appended through an ATM card to a banking customer plugged in from a drive through window, or a patient at an emergency department directly face-to-face with the point of contact provider: the nurse. For better or worse, decisions that mimicked the just-in-time philosophy in the manufacturing and selling of a product were now being applied to the decision-making processes of the professional services delivered by a nurse as front line worker.

Research Versus Evidence-Based Practice

In summary, the quality movement of the eighties brought a new sensibility to nursing research into the early part of the 1990s, to the approaches to quality improvement, and to the use of data or evidence. The intersection of these three dimensions suggested the need for a distinction between research and evidence-based practice, with the latter seen as the new, everyday fare of teams in health care organizations.

This refocused effort brought nurses to the flip chart, and teams could be observed staring at the graphs of dubious yet concrete numbers that indicated an increase or decrease in some purported set of variables of interest. The debates about what a quality initiative was, what did not meet the criteria of research, and what evidence-based practice actually meant were core issues that distinguished these from each other. That is, for the research minded, the traditional route of generating findings for the sake of generating knowledge was one thing. But to articulate, deliver, and evaluate concrete practices that would lead to concrete evidence was another (McSherry, Simmons, Abbott, 2002). If these results could be combined with other studies' results, in systematic reviews, called meta-analysis, all the better. And if these studies and their clear evidence could be documented and placed in easy-to-read formats, then the chances would be enhanced of using the results in places far removed from the location of the original study, and at a cost and in a manner acceptable to the user.

1990 AND BEYOND

By the mid 1990s, the term evidence-based practice began to appear in the health care literature (Stetler, Brunell, Giuliano, Morsi, Prince, & Newell-Stokes, 1998). The Agency for Health Care Policy and Research (AHCPR) coined the term and created steps that would help researchers identify health care initiatives for specific clinical conditions. Subsequently, an epistemological debate took place about evidence-based practice as a viable construct. Its origins and precursors, as shown above, were derived from a variety of sources that include professional practice, research findings, information technology, and managed care (French, 2002). This consideration of evidence-based practice as a viable construct or as a process, French observed, was questionable, and he suggested that no evidence exists to support the notion of "evidence" as a stable construct. Further, he questioned whether or not evidence-based practice is a distinct process, a political construction, or simply another iteration of quality. Several meanings have been associated with the term, and the challenge was to distinguish the practice from personal, subjective informed perception or opinion (French, p. 255).

Opportunities and Challenges

Throughout the 1990s, nursing continued as a major force (Prescott, 1993), as a major cost center, and as a national resource that demanded funding. Nurses understood well and promoted graduate programs that examined the front line bedside nurse as decision-maker, all the more powerful given the ever-expanding integrated health care systems spread over multi-mile campuses. Decision-making, George (1999) argued, belonged at the local level, with the bedside nurse, and interventions now had to lead to evidence to meet the 24-hour turn-around for an overnight hospital stay. Babies and mothers bonded in one day through some miraculous process that used to take several days, weeks, or months. Intensive psychotherapy that once took a lifetime was now reduced to 12 sessions of cognitive therapy and a book that helped the depressed through a 10-step process of recovery. Some confrontation, a book on the topic of angst, and some generic, anti-depressant medication became the silver bullet for providing "mental health services."

In nursing during these years, the discipline's literature databases had extensively documented the empirical, positivist approach to research and simultaneously embraced the post-modern, post-empirical studies that acknowledged the interaction of the researcher with the researched. These qualitative studies questioned our underlying assumptions of the processes that occurred when people, despite all odds, did not die, but flourished. They examined the place of action research, the imperative of which was to alter the research processes to accommodate changes that occurred during the life of the research study, and put reputations at risk as researchers conducted studies that would suggest the relationship between getting well and experiencing music and art as part of the caring process. These qualitative studies appeared in peer-reviewed journals in nursing and were also appearing in what some would characterize as enlightened journals in medicine.

Thus, shortly after appearing in the literature, evidence-based practice, like its predecessors TQM and CQI, had its critics. Some, including Mitchell (1997), suggested that after 50 years of nursing research, little direction was forthcoming in helping nurses enhance patients' quality of life and help them deal with the human responses of loss, despair, and suffering. Not only were the studies conducted at that time perceived as unhelpful, but the move to evidence-based practice, Mitchell asserted, removes the individual approach to participation between the patient and the nurse (p. 154). Evidence-based practice, she said, may call for "decontextualized, menu driven directives based on diagnoses or generalized situations" (p. 155). Yet the characteristic of generalizability is acknowledged as the very goal of evidence-based practice, so that research results can be used in other places without the arduous task of conducting the research again.

These debates and the data generated, as might be predicted, continued to produce mixed sentiments. Some asserted that evidence-based practice was not new as nurses, at the time, had been doing this for years. DiCenso, Cullum, and

Ciliska (1998) examined the major constraints raised within nursing. As with other innovations, its definition was questioned (so vague as to be meaningless), its theoretical source was questioned (the framework lacked scientific verification), its methods (randomized control trials) were narrow in focus, and its sampling frames (with narrow inclusion criteria) were restrictive for generalization to large mixed groups of patients (Deaton, 2001). And researchers, as data collectors, were promoting cookbook nursing.

These perceived drawbacks of evidence-based practice were compounded by the nursing research environment, which presented with its own constraints. Specifically, the environments in which nurses worked were such that the staff could not access research data. Nurses found nursing research theories at an unhelpful level of abstraction, and they experienced a disconnection between the ways results were presented and the ways in which the lives of their patients and their illnesses remained unexamined (DiCenso et al., 1998; McCaughan, Thompson, Cullum, Sheldon, & Thompson, 2002).

Thus, despite the advances in nursing research over the previous 20 years, some asserted that much of the research went unused for a variety of reasons and was classified as "barriers to research utilization" (Funk, Champagne, Tornquist, & Wiese, 1995). These included heavy workloads, aspects of the setting, nurse's lack of time (Ervin, 2002; Funk et al., Wallin, Bostrom, Wikblad, & Ewald, 2003), awareness of and access to research to alter practice (Ervin), nurses' isolation from knowledgeable colleagues (Funk et al.), inability to translate research into practice (Ervin), and feeling incapable of understanding the implications for practice (Funk et al.).

Nurses, however, were not the only disenfranchised group. Patients and their families throughout the country struggled to make sense of the health care system they felt did not listen to them, did not understand them, did not teach them about their health condition, and had no time for them. In the United States, Hillary Clinton heard these concerns and emerged as the champion of health care reform. While Ms. Clinton stomped through the country listening to the horror stories of health care needs gone unattended, Health Ministries in the rest of the world watched and vowed to go their own ways.

Europe continued to push for PHC and the avoidance, at all costs, of becoming like the U.S. health care system. The World Bank funded privatization and the U.S. Agency for International Development (USAID) sponsored projects in Eastern Europe and elsewhere that would spur private practice among physicians and nurses. (Never mind that most Eastern European citizens did not have the wherewithal to pay for private services, and entire health care systems in Eastern Europe, Africa, and Asia were based on a totally different set of assumptions about health and health care delivery.) If these conditions were not enough, the resurgence of other factors would exacerbate the situation.

The world was under siege as populations now lived within the infectious disease era, the chronic disease era, and the social health era. Large populations experienced the resurgence of tuberculosis and bacterial infections, the costly, long-term chronic illnesses of heart disease, cancer, and HIV, *and* the emerging social conditions of drug abuse, adolescent unwed pregnancy, and gang behavior. By this time, the populations of India and China passed the billion marks in population. Thus, for good reason, the search to determine the health care practices that were and were not effective became the imperative on the minds of most concerned governments. Yet progress was slow.

The Language and Alignment of Nursing

Evers (2001) suggests that the purported slow rate of progress to move to evidence-based practice had to do with the congruence between nursing terminology and the terminology of the health community. He argued for a better fit, for example, between the *WHO International Classification of Impairments, Disabilities and Handicaps* (ICIDH) (1980), which asserts the classification not of disease but rather the consequences of disease (Evers, p. 138), and other nomenclatures. He noted the similarity of this nomenclature with Orem's inability for self-care, and Henderson's focus on health deviations and self care requisites. These observations underscored his bid for collaboration among researchers and the developers of taxonomies, and for classifications that document nursing practices, interventions, and outcomes. They also underscore the need for centers of excellence to develop guidelines for these conditions, described as occurring through a process of research utilization (Stetler et al., 1998).

Theories in Use

Other arguments challenge the uptake of evidence-based practice. A major reason, some assert, is that nursing theories provide an abstract view of nursing (Evers, 2001) that appears as generic statements that are at odds with the highly specific results produced through evidence-based practice guidelines and experimental studies that explicate targeted evidence for narrowly defined conditions. This may be due, in part, to the restricted inclusion and exclusion criteria that studies adopt so that, in fact, the results do emerge as clear evidence. However, the specificity of the targeted study subjects precludes the application of the results to large, homogeneous groups of patients and demands a sophisticated reader of research results.

Researchers have conducted studies to examine nurses' clinical decision-making and to identify the sources of information and other enhancers they have found useful in reducing the uncertainty associated with their clinical decisions (Nagy, Lumby, McKinley, & Macfarlane, 2001). In one study, researchers examined the commentaries of 108 nurses in three large acute hospitals in England (Thompson, McCaughan, Thompson, Cullum, Sheldon, Mulhall, & Thompson, 2002). They found that for information to be useful, it had to provide direction, experiential knowledge, organization support for practice, and a combination of research technology and experience. Further, these researchers identified the overwhelming support for human information sources, namely, in the role of the clinical nurse specialist (CNS), whom they characterized as having extensive networks and clinical and research expertise. Importantly, nursing textbooks and information files were not found to be particularly useful. They concluded that research knowledge is not the issue, or the problem; rather the core element is the medium through which research knowledge is delivered (Thompson et al.).

These findings may be generalizable only to the United Kingdom, but hospitals in the United States have begun hiring nurses with titles addressing evidence-based practice, and nursing administrators are extending their support and expectations for research-based nursing delivery to evidence-based practices. Like other innovations, evidence-based practice must meet the criteria for adoption. These criteria are what USAID suggests are requisite qualities of an innovation: it is sustainable, has absorptive capacity, and can be transferable. That is, the efforts can be maintained after initial seed money has been spent; the organization can integrate the materials, concepts, and actions into its existing systems; and the ideas, framework, and practices can be applied in other than the test sites. To ensure meeting these criteria; health care organizations are orienting nurse leaders; hiring, retraining, and renaming CNSs as Specialists for Evidence Based Practice (Stetler et al., 1998); and developing processes, work groups, and data collection instruments to implement the innovations.

A NEW MILLENNIUM

The end of the 20th century came and went, and by any measure, the world did not achieve Health for All. In fact, some would assert, the world's scorecard for health was worse than it had been a decade earlier. One factor that, in part, underscored this status was the move of the public debate on health care to center stage, highlighting the cost of health care, and the disappointing health indicators in the United States, despite the money invested (15% of the gross national product). Some countries with far less resources managed to achieve far better scores on the major indicators of a community's and nation's health status: the under five, infant, and neonatal mortality rates.

In the meantime, insurers, drug companies, health maintenance organizations, physician groups, and individual practices have undergone major changes. Physician groups now specialize in product lines that bring them superior incomes, insurance companies insure the healthy, and consumers have moved to the Internet for information, consolation, and support of groups of like-minded folks who share their illnesses and can at least discuss among *themselves* what they thought they ought to be talking over with their *health care providers*.

Consumers are becoming sophisticated in the ways of their bodies. We debate the opportunities and risks of over-the-counter medications, Canadian drug prices, and the interaction effects of herbs and food supplements on longevity. Huge patient samples in longitudinal investigations yield data in mega-research studies where data are crunched by laptop computers the size of telephones. The Genome Project has erupted onto interconnected computer systems, and Dolly, the sheep that was cloned, has since died.

Thus, while remarkable advances have occurred, political and other forces continue to blind the world to obvious issues that have profound effects on populations. The AIDS epidemic has eliminated entire populations in Africa, while people with AIDS in America have not succumbed after all. Now, a quarter of a century later, AIDS is a chronic illness and those with it are living long lives along with the survivors of cancer, the trisomies, and many other illnesses that a century ago would have spelled almost immediate death. Paradoxically, the illnesses that all thought were under wraps have made their way back into public consciousness. As noted earlier, tuberculosis and other bacterial, viral, and infectious diseases have returned, along with the emotional conditions exacerbated by family and community violence and the ever-impending threat of terrorism.

These remarkable events have affected every part of our lives. They have focused our attention on the brevity of life, the vulnerability of entire nations, and the staggering, domino effects of catastrophic events on a region's physical, social, financial, and community structures. Thus, while the creativity, energy, and intelligence of so many have brought about mind boggling changes to our everyday lives, the seduction persists to find silver bullets for what were, in earlier times, formidable challenges for even the bravest of hearts.

While conceptual models, theories, methods, data collection instruments, Web sites, and Call-a-Nurse services are more available than ever, more nurses than ever are being asked to find the answers in highly specialized databases that extend to infinity through a computerized, World Wide Web that continues to expand beyond what only 15 years ago was unheard of. These same nurses, mostly women, are working 12-hour shifts, supported by an army of traveling nurses, and absorbing the ever-present threats of litigation as clinical areas become increasingly complex.

Nurses in this new century are tempted with generous sign-on bonuses, and baccalaureate graduates are being asked to teach undergraduate students who, a year before, were their college chums. What ordinarily took a fairly long career path is now considered a novice-to-expert trajectory that can be taught in a fraction of the time ordinarily required of most mortal nurses.

Yet the sophistication of computers and the dazzling array of techniques available to researchers require quite the opposite sort of context, thinking frame, and creativity that are not particularly fostered in today's health care environment. In fact, the often slogging, deliberate, obsessive nature of the research process leaves many nurses tiptoeing out of the computer room. The decision-making exercise involved in developing an internally coherent piece of research is, indeed, painstakingly slow and simply does not lend itself to a linear process. On the contrary, a research study in the making is messy, internally incoherent, and at least for a time, nonlinear; it tests the mettle of even the most patient of scientists.

In short, the very evidence to inform practice in this fast-paced, high-risk environment of nursing is found in the data derived from this deliberate, sometimes obscure process of research. And having to read and use the results of research is sometimes as painful as having to carry out the needed study.

All of these contemporary issues in this new millennium serve to focus our attention on the practices that help us to sort out our practices in the shortest amount of time with the maximum of benefit and with the least cost—again not unlike the very characteristics promoted in the Alma Ata Declaration.

Ongoing Tensions

Clearly, the often-voiced impediments to evidence-based practice are powerful. But they pale in the realization that practices are sorely needed that are based on sound evidence and can be carried out with fewer and fewer resources. Thus, the tensions persist between this imperative and the worry that the adoption of evidence-based practice would lead to regimentation (Winch et al., 2002) and government control.

Australian nurse researchers contextualize the concern over evidence-based practice within the framework of Foucault's concept of govenmentality (Winch et al., 2002). That is, Foucault views science as a form of social control through discipline and normalization. For nursing, practitioners can now conduct systematic reviews, cull and rank evidence, create practice guidelines, determine which interventions work and don't work, and identify the research that is needed. The government can then determine the programs types of thought and action that seek to guide their conduct (Cochrane, 1989; cited in Winch et al.). Likewise, the interventions that do not lend themselves to scientific evidence are discounted and a form of rationing results. These authors suggest that this kind of development might also coincide with a loss of nursing's rich intuitive base. Further, the narrow range of research methods, including the randomized control trials and other empirical methods, would preclude the methodological pluralistic approach seen as prohibitively costly. Most importantly, in the Foucaultian framework, a potential exists to influence nurses politically and personally. To counter this possibility, the Australians invite nurses to reframe and reshape the "truth taxonomies" (Winch et al., p. 160) they cherish and to sustain their ability to preserve the intuitive experiences that are a central part of nursing practice.

THE WAY FORWARD

The new millennium and the creativity of nursing has led to ways of distinguishing research from evidence-based practice, and it has begun to provide the structure, processes, mechanisms, and documentation to promote its development. This creative process is spurred on by two major imperatives: the genuine concern for the patient and the pressure to ensure competent care. Each of the challenges raised in the mid and late nineties continues to be addressed.

Now, a new era has brought innovation and an insistence on not doing "what other men have done." Just a few years from its inception, three models of research utilization relate to evidence-based practice in nursing. These are the Conduct and Utilization of Research in Nursing (CURN) Project, the Stetler Model of Research Utilization, and the Iowa Model for Research in Practice (http://www.enursescribe.com/ebnart.htm) (Sisk, 2002). Other advances have occurred as well.

Ervin (2002) has established an Organizational Model of Evidence-Based Practice, and physicians, who coined the term "Evidence-Based Medicine," have developed a journal with the same moniker. The United Kingdom has developed the journal, *Evidence-Based Nursing: Linking Research to Practice*, and Sigma Theta Tau has created the *Online Journal of Knowledge Synthesis for Nursing International*.

Centers have developed, and library and information literacy skills have appeared to strengthen those interested in evidence-based approaches to nursing practice (Shorten, Wallace, Crookes, 2001), and librarians have harnessed their skills to develop a curriculum integrated model to produce "research connoisseurs" (Shorten et al., p. 87). Excellence in evidence-based practice is a hall-mark of nursing practice in the United States, Canada, the United Kingdom, Germany, New Zealand, Germany, and Australia (Sisk, 2002).

The Cochrane Collaboration (Fullerton-Smith, 1995) in England has developed *The Online Journal of Knowledge Synthesis*, and the Cochrane Library has developed holdings of randomized controlled and clinical trials (French, 2002).

Researchers have developed data collection instruments and protocols to examine the differences between evidence-based nursing and evidence-based medicine. Specifically, two scales are available: The Evidence-Based Nursing Scale (Lavin, Meyer, Krieger, McNary, Carlson, Perry, James, & Civitan, 2002) and the Contribution to Nursing Scale. Protocol development is ongoing through the CURN Project, Conduct and Utilization of Research in Nursing, funded by the Division of Nursing, U.S. Department of Health Education and Welfare, under the auspices of the Michigan Nurses Association.

Grossman and Bautista (2002) offer approaches to developing evidence-based nursing protocols; universities are now offering courses and workshops face-to-face and online to train educators in teaching evidence-based clinical practice (How to teach evidence-based clinical practice, 2004), and Health Links, an Internet resource the University of Washington, provides an impressive list of resources on the topic. Some of these include: Meta-search engines, evidence guidelines, clinical research critiques, case report/series/practice guidelines, evidence-based statistics, research centers' calculators, and literature (http://healthlinks.washington.edu/ebp).

EPIDEMIOLOGY OF EVIDENCE-BASED PRACTICE

To date, evidence-based practice has followed its epidemiological path and has undergone definition (AHCPR), the aim of which is to distinguish it from other kinds of activities, including research, to harness the methods that best address it, and to undergo pilot testing. It is now being applied in a variety of settings. To ensure this trajectory, researchers, health care providers, librarians, and information technology specialists have established these journals, programs, data collection instruments, and protocols, and centers of excellence in various parts of the world. Further, they have specified the phenomenon of interest—evidence-based practice—underway with the launching of this text. This emerging phenomenon is expanding as it addresses ways to manage the information infrastructure, education, outcome management, workload management, legislation, systems development, leadership, and healing—the very elements that formed the structure of this text and the living evidence that supports research into practice—evidence-based practice, that is.

REFERENCES

Cochrane, A. L. (1989). Effectiveness and efficiency: Random reflections on the health service. *Controlled Clinical Trials, 10*(4), 428–433.

Deaton, C. (2001). Outcomes measurement and evidence-based nursing practice. *Journal of Cardiovascular Nursing, 15*(2), 83–86.

Deming, W. E. (2000). *Out of the Crisis.* Cambridge, MA: Massachusetts Institute of Technology.

DiCenso, A., Cullum, N., & Ciliska, D. (1998). Implementing evidence-based nursing: Some misconceptions. *Evidence-Based Nursing, 1,* 38–40. Available at http://ebn.bmjjournals.com. Retrieved February 17, 2005.

Donabedian, A. (1980). *Explorations in Quality Assessment and Monitoring.* Ann Arbor, MI: Health Administration Press.

Donabedian, A. (1988). The quality of care: How can it be defined? *Journal of the American Medical Association, 260*(12), 1743–1748.

Ervin, N. E. (2002). Evidence-based nursing practice: Are we there yet? *Journal of the New York State Nurses Association, 33*(2), 11–16.

Evers, G. C. M. (2001). Naming nursing: Evidence-based nursing. *Nursing Diagnosis, 12*(4), 137–142.

Farrell, M. (Ed). (1987a). *People's Needs for Nursing Care: A European Study.* Copenhagen: European Regional Office, World Health Organization.

Farrell, M. (Ed). (1987b). *Nursing Care: Summary of a European Study.* Copenhagen: World Health Organization.

Foss, S. W. (1911). *The Calf-Path.* From http://www.giga-usa.com/gigaweb1/quotes2/qutopprecedentx001.htm. Retrieved May 21, 2005.

French, P. (2002). What is the evidence on evidence-based nursing? An epistemological concern. *Journal of Advanced Nursing, 37*(3), 250–257.

Fullerton-Smith, I. (1995). How members of the Cochrane Collaboration prepare and maintain systematic reviews of the effects of health care. *Evidence-Based Medicine, 1*:7–8.

Funk, S. G., Champagne, M. T., Tornquist, E. M., & Wiese, R. A. (1995). Administrators' views on barriers to research utilization. *Applied Nursing Research, 8*(1), 44–49.

George, V. (1999). *An Organizational Case Study of Shared Leadership Development in Nursing.* (Unpublished doctoral dissertation, Marquette University, 1999).

Goldratt, E. M., & Fox, R. E. (1986). *The Race.* Crotonon-Hudson, NY: North Rivers Press.

Grossman, S., & Bautista, C. (2002). Collaboration yields cost-effective, evidence-based nursing protocols. *Orthopaedic Nursing, 21*(3), 30–36.

How to teach evidence-based clinical practice. (2004). McMaster University Workshop. Available at http://www.cche.net/ebcp/info.asp. Retrieved on February 17, 2005.

International Classification of Impairments, Disabilities, and Handicaps. (1980). Geneva: World Health Organization.

Juran, J. M. (1989). *Juran on Leadership for Quality: An Executive Handbook.* New York: The Free Press.

Juran, J. M. (1992). *Juran on Quality by Design.* New York: The Free Press.

Lavin, M. A., Meyer, G., Krieger, M., McNary, P., Mals, R. N., Carlson, J., Perry, A., James, D., & Civitan, T. (2002). Essential differences between evidence-based nursing and evidence-based medicine. *International Journal of Nursing Terminologies and Classifications, 12*(3), 101–106.

McCaughan, D., Thompson, C., Cullum, N., Sheldon, T. A., & Thompson, D. R. (2002). Acute care nurses' perceptions of barriers to using research information in clinical decision-making. *Journal of Advanced Nursing, 39*(1), 46–60.

McSherry, R., Simmons, M., & Abbott, P. (2002). *Evidence-Informed Nursing: A Guide for Clinical Nurses.* London: Routledge.

Mitchell, G. J. (1997). Questioning evidence-based practice for nursing. *Nursing Science Quarterly, 10*(4), 154–155.

Nagy, S., Lumby, J., McKinley, S., & Macfarlane, C. (2001). Nurses' beliefs about the conditions that hinder or support evidence-based nursing. *International Journal of Nursing Practice, 7*(5), 314–321.

Parker, J. (2002). Evidence based nursing: A defence. *Nursing Inquiry, 9*(3), 139–140.

Pirzig, R. L. (1991). *Lila: An Inquiry of Morals.* New York: Bantam Books.

Prescott, P. (1993). Nursing: An important component of hospital survival under a reformed health care system. *Nursing Economic$, 11*(4), 192–199.

Primary Health Care. (1978). (Alma Ata, 1978). Health for All Series No.1. Geneva: World Health Organization. www.euro.who.int/AboutWHO/Policy/20010827_1.

Shilts, R. (1987). *And the Band Played On.* New York: Bedford/St. Martins Press.

Shorten, A., Wallace, M. S., & Crookes, P. A. (2001). Developing information literacy: A key to evidence-based nursing. *International Nursing Review, 48*, 86–92.

Sisk, B. (2002). Evidence-based nursing. Available at http://www.enursescribe.com/ebnart.htm. Retrieved February 17, 2005.

Stetler, C. B., Brunell, M., Giuliano, K. K., Morsi, D., Prince, L., & Newell-Stokes, V. (1998). Evidence-based practice and the role of nursing leadership. *Journal of Nursing Administration, 28*(7/8), 45–53.

Targets for HFA. (1991). Copenhagen: World Health Organization European Regional Office.

Tarimo, E., Cresse, A. (1990). Achieving Health for All by the Year 2000: Midway Reports Country Experiences. Geneva: WHO.

Thompson, C., McCaughan, D., Thompson, C., Cullum, N., Sheldon, T. A., & Thompson, D. R. (2002). Research information in nurses' clinical decision-making: What is useful? *Journal of Advanced Nursing, 36*(3), 376 http://www.enursescribe.com/ebnart.htm.

University of Washington. Evidence-based practice. Health links. Available at http://healthlinks.washington.edu/ebp. Retrieved February 17, 2005.

Wallin, L., Bostrom, A. M., Wikblad, K., & Ewald, U. (2003). Sustainability in changing clinical practice promotes evidence-based nursing care. *Journal of Advanced Nursing, 41*(5), 509–518.

Winch, S., Creedy, D., & Chaboyer, W. (2002). Governing nursing conduct: The rise of evidence-based practice. *Nursing Inquiry, 9*(3), 156–161.

CHAPTER 6

The Journey to Evidence: Managing the Information Infrastructure

Robert C. Geibert

The diffusion of technology into the health care system and, in particular, incorporating the powers of the Internet are perhaps the most significant factors in supporting and developing the integration of evidence-based practice (EBP) into the provision of patient care. With 24/7 access to clinical data, clinicians can search for information from a growing number of online resources sponsored by organizations worldwide and incorporate findings into their clinical decision-making process. The availability of electronic networks provides access to data at the point of care, whether it is the clinic exam room, the hospital bedside, or at a patient's home. It is no longer necessary to visit a medical library during hours of operation to find answers to clinical questions. This chapter discusses how the integration of technology and enhanced access to data can support EBP and thereby improve patient care.

Health care practitioners are not the only beneficiaries of this wealth of information. Health care consumers—our patients—also can access a significant amount of health-related data via the Internet at sites like WebMD (http://www.webmd.com), Mayo Clinic (http://www.mayoclinic.com), and the Johns Hopkins Hospital and Health System (http://www.hopkinshospital.org/health_info). According to Nielsen//NetRatings as reported by Robyn Greenspan (2004), in June 2004 the United States had 138,805,566 active Internet users as defined by the number of people that actually go online in a given month. A recent study (Fox & Fallows, 2003) reported that 52 million Americans access health or medical information on the Web. The National Library of Medicine's MEDLINE is accessed by consumers as frequently as by health care professionals and researchers (Thompson & Brailer, 2004). Thus, the number of consumers who have access to public online health-related sites is significant and enables them to be better informed participants regarding their care.

As our health care system continues to advance, technology will play an ever increasing role in its expansion. The Honorable Tommy Thompson, former U.S. Health and Human Services Secretary, at the July 2004 Secretarial Summit on Health Information Technology stated, "our health care system needs all the help it can get, and health information technology is the best medicine we can get" (Beck, 2004). On July 21, 2004, Mr. Thompson's office released a report prepared by David J. Brailer, the new National Coordinator for Health Information Technology (Thompson & Brailer, 2004) that laid out the broad steps needed to achieve always-current, always-available, electronic health records for Americans.

As the title suggests, the report provides a vision for consumer-centric and information-rich care. It envisions the following:

- Medical information will follow the consumer
- Information tools will guide medical decisions
- Clinicians will have appropriate access to a patient's complete treatment history, medical records, medication history, and laboratory and radiographic results
- Computerized medication orders will eliminate handwriting errors, automatically check for doses that are too high or too low, check for harmful drug-drug interactions, and check for allergies
- Prescriptions will be checked against a health plan's formulary, and out-of-pocket costs can be compared with alternative treatments
- Electronic alerts will remind clinicians about treatment procedures and medical guidelines

Systems such as these are available now and are being implemented in organizations around the world. It is clear that technology is a significant, and perhaps a deciding, factor in the ability of organizations to provide evidence-based methodologies for their clinicians.

THE ELECTRONIC HEALTH RECORD

The electronic health record (EHR) is known by many names. Some more common ones are: computer-based patient record, electronic medical record, and automated medical record. EHR is used here because it is consistent with the U.S. Department of Health and Human Services terminology in reference to its Framework for Strategic Action. In addition, "EHR is believed to represent the most comprehensive vision of an information system that would support all types of caregivers, in all settings, including the individual who may be using it to record personal health status information" (Amatayakul, 2004, p. 6).

Many factors affect the integration of technology into health care environments. A study done by the Medical Records Institute in 2002 (Brailer & Terasawa, 2003) found that factors to increase adoption fell into two categories: (a) administrative, and (b) clinical. Major administrative drivers as reported by the percentage of respondents were:

- Need to share comparable patient data among different sites within a multi-entity health care delivery system (74.7%)
- Need to improve clinical documentation to support appropriate billing service levels (75.3%)
- Requirement to contain or reduce health care delivery costs (66.3%)
- Need to establish a more efficient and effective information infrastructure as a competitive advantage (64.3%)
- Need to meet the requirements of legal, regulatory, or accreditation standards (60.4%)
- Need to manage capitation contracts (21.8%)

Major clinical factors that drive EHR adoption are

- Improve the ability to share patient record information among health care practitioners and professionals within the enterprise (90%)
- Improve quality of care (85.3%)
- Improve clinical processes or workflow efficiency (83.8%)
- Improve clinical data capture (82.6%)
- Reduce medical errors (increase patient safety; 81.9%)
- Provide access to patient records at remote locations (70.9%)
- Facilitate clinical decision support (70.4%)
- Improve employee/physician satisfaction (62.8%)
- Improve patient satisfaction (60.2%)
- Improve efficiency via pre-visit health assessments and post-visit patient education (39.9%)
- Support and integrate patient health care information from Web-based personal health records (30.3%)
- Retain health plan membership (8.5%)

A recent Medical Records Institute survey (2004) found that the factors driving the need for EHR systems included:

- The need to improve clinical processes or workflow efficiency (85%)
- The need to improve quality of care (83%)
- The need to share patient record information among health care practitioners (80%)
- The need to improve patient safety by reducing medical errors (76%)

Geography and the size of health care organizations also impact the implementation of EHRs (Brailer & Terasawa). They reported that adoption in major metropolitan areas was 1.5 times greater than in small non-urban markets. They further suggested that organizational size appeared to influence the adoption of EHRs and found that large hospitals had an electronic capture of 30% more information than small hospitals. They posited that large organizations had an advantage in all aspects of the information technology implementation lifecycle, including planning, financing, acquiring, installing, implementing, and supporting the systems. Their study also noted that smaller organizations often do not have the resources to invest in, implement, or operate the complicated infrastructures that are required for an EHR.

Unfortunately, the integration of technology into health care systems lags behind most other industries. According to the HHS Fact Sheet (2004), hospitals' use of EHRs in 2002 was reported at 13%; and for physicians' practices, from 14% to a possible high of 28%. In comparison, it is common to find an automated veterinarian office that, with the press of a few keys, can prepare and send out personalized reminders when vaccinations or other procedures are due for our pets. How often do we receive preventive care reminders from our clinicians' offices?

Consumers are becoming accustomed to receiving personalized service that is supported by technology. For example, after using an online retailer such as Amazon (http://www.amazon.com), the consumer is welcomed back with customer-focused suggestions based upon past purchases or profiles. What a contrast to the more familiar visit to the medical clinic where, even with an appointment, the chart is not available when the patient arrives, and the clinician must make decisions with limited, or perhaps even incorrect patient or caregiver-provided information.

BARRIERS TO EHR ADOPTION

EHRs are technologically complex and very expensive applications to implement. They also require significant change within an organization. Thus, there are many barriers to adoption. The following section examines some of these barriers.

Funding, resource availability, and lack of support are the largest barriers to EHR adoption regardless of the organization's size. A 2004 MRI survey found that lack of resources was cited as the top barrier by 55.5% of respondents. Lack of support by medical staff was reported by 35.4% of those responding.

A 2002 Sheldon Dorenfest study (Brailer, 2003) reviewed hospital spending on information technology as a percent of their budgets, and found that 44% of hospitals spent less than 2% of their budgets on information technology, and 93% spent less than 4%. In addition, only 7% of hospitals spent 4% or more of their budgets on information technology. Some respondents suggested that a 7% expenditure is the threshold that must be met to accommodate rapid information technology adoption in hospitals. In summary, the data suggest that organizations must significantly increase their contributions to health information technology to be able to take advantage of the benefits an EHR provides.

Although the financial expenditures required to implement health information technology are significant, organizations must hold the perception that the expenditure will be valuable. The HHS report (Thompson & Brailer) included an interesting comparison between the value of magnetic resonance imaging (MRI) and the EHR. Both technologies collect a variety of data, summarize data with algorithms, store and communicate data, and present data in a manner that is meaningful to clinicians. Both provide information that supplements diagnostic decision-making. Like MRIs, EHRs are expensive to purchase and operate, and their payback period is extended. In contrast, however, this study pointed out that EHRs are different from an MRI machine in one notable way: EHRs evolved from an administrative to a clinical tool. When clinicians experience the power and value of EHRs, and how electronic clinical decision support systems can enhance the care they provide to their patients, the move to technology-assisted care will accelerate. Much like the MRI, the EHR will increasingly be perceived as an indispensable clinical tool.

CLINICAL INFORMATION-SEEKING NEEDS

When considering the adoption of an EHR to improve patient care and clinical decision-making, it would be prudent to examine the information-seeking needs of clinicians. The research in this area is limited, although informative. Research indicates that internal medicine clinicians needed clinical information approximately twice for every three patients seen (Covell, Uman, & Manning, 1985). A 1995 study found that rates of information needs varied from 0.013 to 5.044 questions per patient encounter (D'Alessandro, Kreiter, & Peterson, 2004).

Information resources at the point of care have a positive impact on clinical decision-making. For example, drug-allergy or drug-drug interactions can be avoided when prescribing medications. Unfortunately, there are numerous obstacles to accessing information, and the lack of time is one of the most common (D'Alessandro et al., 2004; Ely, Osheroff, Ebell, Chambliss, Vinson, & Stevermer, 2002). Other obstacles (Osheroff, 1991) include a lack of knowledge about appropriate answer sources, and a reliance on convenient information sources, even when more appropriate resources were available. According to Ely et al., clinicians found inadequate synthesis of multiple bits of evidence that were presented in a clinically useful statement.

It is not surprising that information is difficult to find, because the amount of clinical information that is available is exploding. The National Library of Medicine indexes approximately 500,000 articles annually to add to the MEDLINE database (Fact sheet, 2003). These new items are added to the existing 11 million articles from approximately 4,600 of the world's preeminent biomedical journals that have been indexed since 1966.

Because of the enormous amount of information available, it is increasingly difficult for health care providers to remain current. Research has shown that physicians incorporate the latest medical evidence into their treatment decisions about 50% of the time (McGlynn et al., 2003). When identifying a gap in knowledge, clinicians must decide whether to do the best they can with their current knowledge, or to expand that knowledge by formulating and answering a question (Ely et al.). In a busy work environment, doing the best one can is often the only practical approach. This finding is not limited to health care environments. Any worker in an occupation that is dependent upon on-demand information to perform the duties of their work experiences similar challenges. Rae and O'Driscoll (2004) refer to information availability as "proximity," and to the likelihood that what is provided will meet the needs of the information seeker as "relevancy." Providing clinical decision support systems (CDSSs) that are easily accessible and reliable is a strong contributing factor that may encourage clinicians to seek information to unanswered questions, rather than relying on their current knowledge.

CLINICAL DECISION SUPPORT SYSTEMS

Many clinicians are familiar with computer systems that manage laboratory data, and pharmacy systems that track prescriptions and refills. As they become accustomed to searching for and displaying data with the press of a few keys, it is unlikely that they will want to return to the often tedious task of shuffling papers to find individual pieces of data.

Although EHRs can capture, transform, display, and analyze some data, they may not filter and abstract information to the extent needed for complex decision-making. CDSSs take this one step further. As detailed individual patient data are input into a computer program, they are sorted and matched to programs or algorithms in a computerized knowledge base, resulting in the generation of patient-specific assessments or recommendations for clinicians (Randolph, Haynes, Wyatt, Cook, & Guyatt, 2001). Wyatt and Spiegelhalter, as reported by

Johnston et al. (1994), define a clinical-decision support system as an "active knowledge system which use two or more items of patient data to generate case-specific advice." Amatayakul believes that this help is provided at the point of care and can tap external knowledge sources. Computerized management systems are complex, and system-generated suggestions regarding an optional decision are based upon the information currently known by the system (Randolph et al.)

What, then, are the key functions of a CDSS? Table 6.1 outlines a few suggestions from Pryor, as reported by Randolph et al. (2001).

VALUE OF CLINICAL DECISION SUPPORT SYSTEMS

An average of 195,000 people in the United States died due to potentially preventable, in-hospital medical errors in each of the years 2000, 2001, and 2002 according to a new study of 37 million patient records (HealthGrades, 2004). The HealthGrades study found nearly double the number of deaths from medical errors as reported in the 1999 Institute of Medicine study. According to Dr. Samatha Collier, HealthGrades' Vice President of Medical Affairs, "the equivalent of 390 jumbo jets full of people are dying each year due to likely preventable, in-

Table 6.1   Clinical Decision Support System (CDSS)

Function	Example
Alerting	Highlighting out-of-range laboratory values
Reminding	Reminding the clinician to schedule a mammogram
Critiquing	Rejecting an electronic order
Interpreting	Interpreting the electrocardiogram
Predicting	Predicting risk of mortality from a severity of illness score
Diagnosing	Listing a differential diagnosis for a patient with chest pain
Assisting	Tailoring the antibiotic choices for liver transplant and renal failure
Suggesting	Generating suggestions for adjusting the mechanical ventilator

hospital medical errors, making this one of the leading killers in the U.S." (Health-Grades, 2004; Underwood, 2004).

A growing field of evidence supports the use of health information technology to enhance patient safety, quality, and continuity of care. Evidence consistently demonstrates that errors can be reduced by the appropriate use of computerized physician provider order entry (CPOE) and decision support systems, particularly in the case of drug prescribing, dispensing, and administration (Thompson & Brailer). The HHS report cites several examples: (1) At the LDS Hospital in Salt Lake City, a CPOE system reduced adverse drug events by 75%; (2) at the Regenstrief Institute for Health Care in Indianapolis, researchers demonstrated that automated computerized reminders increased orders for recommended interventions from 22% to 46%; (3) a 1998 systematic literature review that assessed the effects of 68 computer-based clinical decision support systems demonstrated a beneficial impact on physician performance in 43 of 65 studies, and a beneficial effect on patient outcomes in 6 of 14 studies; and (4) a new pharmacy software system implemented by the Department of Defense in 2001, which integrates and reviews information from all sources prior to prescriptions being filled, has eliminated over 100,000 adverse drug interactions.

Other factors that are influencing the increased implementation of clinical information systems are: (1) greater support from physicians; (2) patient expectations; and (3) improvements in the technology itself (Briggs, 2004). In addition, organizations find that EHRs assist them in more easily collecting and reporting data to meet accrediting body requirements.

TECHNOLOGY AND EVIDENCE-BASED PRACTICE

How does the diffusion of technology into a health care system support evidence-based practice (EBP)? David Sackett, a pioneer in evidence-based medicine (EBM), defines EBM as, "the conscientious, explicit and judicious use of current best evidence in making decisions about the care of individual patients" (Sackett, Rosenberg, Gray, Haynes, & Richardson, 1996). He further states that, "the practice of evidence-based medicine means integrating individual clinical expertise with the best available external clinical evidence from systematic research." A less formal definition is that EBM is a, "bridge between clinical research and clinical practice, bringing the best applicable evidence from scientific research to the provision of patient care" (Kaiser Permanente, 1999).

It is further postulated that technology is the bridge to integrating EBP into patient care. It is the electronic highway that enables information dissemination and access that is neither time-nor place-dependent. It is a lifeline to the external clinical evidence that Sackett describes.

DEVELOPING THE INFRASTRUCTURE

Infrastructure is defined by the American Heritage Dictionary (2001) as "an underlying base, especially for an organization or system." Creating a technologic infrastructure that will support EBP is a challenging undertaking. The first solution that generally comes to mind is to purchase software that will enable the input, storage, and retrieval of data to support clinical decisions. Although this is a critical component, and one that frequently receives the most attention, it is only one piece of the overall structure. Infrastructure has three basic components: (1) strategy; (2) people; and (3) architecture. Without considering and planning for each of these components, organizations run the risk of not achieving their desired outcomes.

The health care literature offers limited guidance on this subject. Although an abundance of resources describe why an integrated, technology-rich health care system is needed, and what challenges an organization may face when implementing technology-based solutions, few provide insight into the systems that must be in place to achieve these goals. Based upon experience in implementing Web-based instruction into organizations, the writer turned to the e-learning literature as a parallel resource, because the goals and challenges are similar, for example, moving from a classroom (paper-based) to an online (technology-based) model.

Hunter Harvey and Geibert (2003) posited that it is important to examine the integration of the Web into organizations from a systemic perspective. This is also true when implementing technologic solutions that support EBP. Some aspects to consider include:

- Rationale: What is the rationale for incorporating technology to support EBP?
- Skill preparedness: Does the organization have human resources ready to support the transition from a paper to electronic world?
- Technology issues: Is a suitable technology infrastructure present to achieve the organizational goals?
- Resistance to change: Are front line implementation resources prepared to make the necessary changes and to accommodate the paradigm shift?
- User preparedness and user support: Is appropriate support available for users?
- Professional development opportunities: Will users receive adequate training to enable them to effectively achieve desired outcomes?
- Technology support: Is 24/7 technology support available? Are the support system personnel conversant with the issues involved with electronic delivery?

It is important for organizations to carefully assess each of these components as they relate to developing an infrastructure to support technology-assisted patient care. Lack of attention to and significant planning for any one of these items will have a negative impact on a successful implementation.

REFRAMING STRATEGIC PLANNING

A strategy is a plan of action. Rosenberg (2001) offers a strategic foundation for e-learning that can be applied to creating a strategy that is applicable to EBP and suggests that we must address:

- A new approach to e-learning: In the health care environment, this can include online training (the instructional strategy) and knowledge management (the informational strategy), which provides informational databases and performance support tools to support EBP.
- Learning architecture: the coordination of e-learning with the rest of the organization's learning efforts. EBP must not be a stand alone project; rather, it must be integrated and coordinated with other initiatives.
- Infrastructure: using the organization's technological capabilities to deliver and manage computerized decision support. Rosenberg suggests that the lack of a good infrastructure can stop e-learning in its tracks. Inadequate or ineffective technology capabilities will, without doubt, negatively impact the implementation of EBP.
- Learning cultures, management ownership, and change management: the creation of an environment that encourages learning as a valuable business activity. The integration of technology and clinical decision support must be perceived as a value within the organization as evidenced by management support.
- Sound business case: one that supports technology-based EBP.
- Reinventing the training organization: the adoption of an organizational and business model that supports EBP.

PLANNING FOR TECHNOLOGY INTEGRATION

Integration of an EHR into an organization is frequently identified as a new technology project on which the organization will embark. Although this is a true statement, the more closely the EHR can be linked to the organization's mission, goals, objectives, and other strategic initiatives, the more likely it will be viewed as an integral part of them (Amatayakul). George (2002) suggested that one of the biggest risks new initiatives face is to become "collateralized." This means that the initiative doesn't become "doing business as usual." Instead, it is seen as a program, or something that is being done with spare time or resources. He noted that failures of previous programs to reach sustainability are a strong paradigm that must be broken. After observing several failed initiatives, the common responses from individuals who were scheduled to use the new systems were, "Here we go again," or "I wonder what the next one will be?" Changing attitudes such as these is extremely difficult and adds to the challenge of ensuring a successful implementation.

Planning strategically, and with infinite detail, is critical to achieving success. Amatayakul (2004) discussed a recent study of chief technology officers that found that 10% did not do strategic planning for technology. Their rationale was that strategic planning was frustrating and time consuming, and interfered with their real work of building and maintaining a technology infrastructure. However, those who were surveyed indicated that good planning did help achieve impressive outcomes and did so with a minimum of frustration.

The respondents are correct. Strategic planning for technology implementations is indeed frustrating and time consuming. This is especially true for EHR implementations because they: (1) are generally among the largest technology integrations that an organization will ever experience; (2) are implemented in phases over an extended period of time; (3) involve and affect multiple departments and people; (4) require substantial financial investments; and (5) require changes in the way business will be done. This is no simple task. However, having a clearly defined strategy and implementation plan will contribute significantly to a successful outcome.

During the strategic planning process, organizations must decide what EHR components will be implemented, and when. For example, EHR functionality ranges from simple to sophisticated and may include: (1) document-scanning/imaging systems; (2) order communication/results retrieval systems; (3) clinical messaging systems; (4) patient care charting; (5) CPOE systems; (6) CDSSs; (7) provider-patient portals; (8) personal health records; and (9) population health (Amatayakul). Although each of these components offers important functionality, most planners will focus on CPOE and CDSS because they are an integral support to EBP.

KNOWLEDGE MANAGEMENT

CDSSs involve KM, which Rosenberg (2001) defined as strategies for delivering knowledge in the digital age. KM supports the "creation, archiving, and sharing of valued information, expertise, and insight within and across communities of people and organizations with similar interests and needs" (p. 66). Rosenberg suggested that KM can be divided into three levels as represented by a pyramid: (1) document management, (2) information creation, sharing, and management, and (3) enterprise intelligence. He also indicates that the KM system is integrated more with actual work the higher that one goes up on the pyramid (Figure 6.1).

Components of an EHR can easily be compared to the KM pyramid. Document management might involve digitized copies of paper documents, for example, signed consents. Data available for access and retrieval might represent laboratory or radiology results. The second level (information creation, sharing, and management) is represented by clinicians contributing information to the system, creating new content, and adding to the data contained in the knowledge database. Examples include: documenting patient encounters, allergies, medications, family and social history, and demographics. Data are easily updated and communicated.

In level three, Rosenberg suggests that the actual operation of the business depends on the expertise that is embedded in the system. People rely upon it in the performance of their jobs, and the resulting experiences are captured and added to the system in a way that increases the collective intelligence of the business. An example of this includes the data that are collected and mined to determine "best practice" interventions in treating certain medical conditions.

Figure 6.1   Knowledge Management (KM) Pyramid

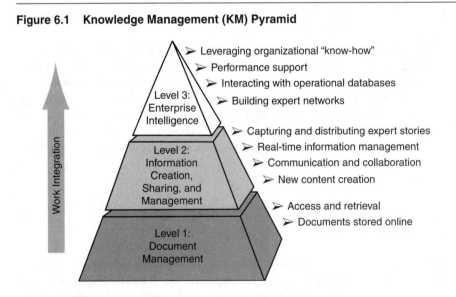

From Rosenberg, *E-Learning: Strategies for Delivering Knowledge in the Digital Age.* (2001). Used with permission from McGraw Hill.

The concept of KM can be easily applied to EHR functionality. Basic EHRs are built upon access, retrieval, and the online storage of documentation. This progresses to a higher level where information is managed in real-time. Finally, the top of the pyramid is represented by EHRs that provide performance support and are built upon expert networks. The next section will explore levels of EHR functionality.

LEVELS OF EHR FUNCTIONALITY

Gartner, Inc. Consulting describes the levels of EHR functionality as "generations" and suggests that implementation follows a migration path (Amatayakul). The five generations are: (1) The Collector, (2) The Documenter, (3) The Helper, (4) The Partner, and (5) The Mentor. Each generation will be described briefly.

Collector Generation

In the Collector generation, systems provide a site-specific, encounter-based solution to accessing clinical data. This is sometimes referred to as results retrieval. This generation does not provide work flow or decision support, no KM is contained, and communications are basically unidirectional. The Collector generation corresponds to Rosenberg's Level 1 of the pyramid, which includes the access of laboratory or radiology results.

Documenter Generation

The Documenter generation is the phase where documentation occurs at the point of care. CPOE with drug-drug and drug-allergy alerts is provided. Minimal access to knowledge sources is available, and communication is simple and bidirectional. Sternlieb (Amatayakul, p. 95) suggests that, "the difficulty in getting CPOE systems adopted is that they lack the decision support capability that would return value to the provider using the system."

Helper Generation

This generation includes more advanced EHR systems that use decision support to assist clinicians and cover episodes and encounters. Documentation functionality, data display, work flow, decision support, and knowledge management are beginning to be integrated, and communication is more complex. According to Amatayakul, Gartner believes that industry is still in the Documenter generation, although it is possible that many organizations are in the Helper generation without the CPOE component.

Partner Generation

The Partner generation includes more complex decision support and encompasses EBM. This generation contains links to personal health records. It is suggested that this level of system is needed to fully support a CPOE. Amatayakul reports that although some organizations have this level of EHR, it is often only in limited areas of the organization.

Mentor Generation

The most complex and sophisticated level is known as the "Mentor" generation, which guides clinicians through highly advanced KM, decision support, and predictive modeling, and is fully integrated across the continuum of care (Amatayakul). This generation benefits from an integrated delivery network with an enterprising master person index. This means that patient data are available in multiple provider settings throughout a health care system. For example, medical offices, clinics, and hospitals in a multi-facility organization will share patient data.

This is the goal of organizations such as the Kaiser Permanente Foundation Health Plan, Inc., which began a corporation-wide EHR program named "Kaiser Permanente HealthConnect." KP HealthConnect, when fully implemented, will provide point-of-care access to the EHR for its more than 11,000 physicians and 8.5 million members. It is also the goal of the United Kingdom's National Institute of Health, which is developing an integrated system that includes electronic records, electronic appointment books, e-prescribing, enhanced Internet broadband capabilities, and expanded personal health care records (Beck).

An EHR implementation can follow many paths. As the EHR functionality includes more features and becomes more complex, the technology and integration of the systems become more sophisticated and challenging. Therefore, each organization should look closely at the specific business needs it is trying to solve, the resources that are available, and plan its strategy carefully. Many organizations respond to these challenges by taking an incremental approach to an EHR migration. They may implement only portions of functionality associated with a particular generation as they transition from a paper-based to an electronic system. Others will implement a particular feature in a higher generation as they are simultaneously completing the integration of a lower generation of functionality.

As was previously stated, an advanced system is required to support complex decision-making activities. Earlier generation document and data retrieval systems provide a valuable resource for clinical decision-making and are where organizations begin in their migration paths. However, the integration of more robust and technology-rich systems must be considered as necessary components to support EBP at its highest level.

People

Another component to consider in this infrastructure is the people who will be involved. Doncaster and Hunter Harvey (2003) refer to this as "peopling" the effort. Implementing an EHR requires a significant investment of human resources that begins many months, if not years, prior to the actual implementation. The need for enhanced levels of human resource will continue throughout—and beyond—the initial implementation as upgrades or additional functionalities are applied. Leaders must be instrumental in shaping organizational culture and obtaining alignment within the organization to ensure that support is available to sustain technology-based initiatives.

Unfortunately, when implementing technologic solutions, it is the technology, rather than the people, that frequently receives the most attention. Admittedly, the "gee whiz" factor is difficult to ignore, as vendors and others demonstrate the products that are to be implemented. However, it is the people who make or break a successful implementation.

As application end users, clinicians will need a new knowledge base and skill sets to enable them to use EHRs effectively. In many cases, however, advances in technology have rapidly outpaced the capabilities of end users to use them effectively. It is a common perception that, in this technological age, everyone knows how to use computers. Unfortunately, this is not true. Although many clinicians are computer savvy and newly graduated clinicians enter the workforce with technology skills, there are large numbers of clinicians who are at best technological novices. Some clinicians will be familiar only with mainframe systems that use keyboards for data entry, and will need to learn how to navigate with a mouse. Others have poor typing skills and cannot document at rates either equal to, or faster than, writing by hand. Still others are computer phobic, and may even consider retiring early or changing to a work environment where the use of technology to complete everyday tasks may not be as integrated into the workflow. Each of these groups deserves attention to achieve a successful implementation.

A recommended activity prior to an EHR implementation is to survey end users regarding their personal computer (PC) skills. These survey results are used to determine how many individuals will need PC training prior to the implementation. Although the results may provide valuable information, they may not be adequate to meet the desired objectives. For example, an EHR trainer reported that when participants entered EHR training, the trainers noted a discrepancy with actual PC skills in comparison to survey results. They found that some respondents overestimated their PC skills, perhaps because they were embarrassed and didn't want others to know that their computer skills were limited. Other respondents underestimated their skills because they thought there would be some aspect of PC knowledge they did not possess and, therefore, thought they would not be able to perform effectively during the EHR implementation.

Because obtaining accurate data was needed to ensure that end users have the requisite PC skills to be successful in an EHR implementation, the trainers contacted department managers for input. In most cases, managers were aware of those individuals who were PC-challenged. In addition, the managers could identify those experienced staff members who were often the individuals that colleagues turned to when computer-related issues arose during the work day. Therefore, a combination of a self-reporting survey coupled with department manager validation may provide more reliable data than by using the survey alone and is highly recommended.

Roles and Responsibilities

It is well-known that establishing clearly defined roles and responsibilities for everyone involved in a project is critical to its success. Although there is great variety among organizations in labeling various roles, I found five roles as described by George (2002) in *Lean Six Sigma* to be a helpful model. He suggests the following structure: (1) Chief Executive Officer (CEO)/President, (2) Business Unit Managers, (3) Line Managers, (4) Champions, and (5) Belts.

CEO/President

This is the person who must decide that adopting the EHR is of strategic importance to the company. He or she must consistently communicate the strategic priorities to the top-level management staff, and to the organization as a whole. Monitoring the project's results, as compared to the plan, and taking corrective action is within this person's realm of responsibility.

Business Unit Manager

These individuals work with the champions to articulate the implementation strategy. They provide input and guidance regarding the EHR functionality that will best support business needs. They also recommend when functionality should be added to the implementation curriculum. The business unit manager works with the champions to (1) identify, develop, and support black belts (George's term for experts) and other resources; (2) create a deployment plan for their unit; (3) solve business problems; and (4) inspire and drive the initiative during the rollout.

Line Manager

Line managers report to a business unit manager and own the processes that will be impacted by the implementation of the EHR. They are sometimes referred to as "process owners." Their specific responsibilities include: (1) aiding in project selection by contributing their intimate knowledge of the processes; (2) contributing to the selection of black belts; (3) creating an environment that will contribute to project success; (4) working with the unit champion and black belts to provide data and insight; (5) monitoring project progress; and (6) sustaining the improvements after black belts move on to another project.

Champions

There are two types of champions: (1) company or group, and (2) business unit. George recommends that company champions should report to the CEO, the Chief Operating Officer (COO), or president. Their roles include: (1) leading the design team; (2) helping to develop the strategy; and (3) monitoring the execution of the project. Their primary responsibility is to ensure that the organization executes a consistent and rapid deployment.

Business unit champions are responsible for: (1) developing the schedule and deployment plans for a unit in conjunction with the unit manager and the implementation team; (2) overseeing the deployment in their business unit; (3) providing communication and ensuring that best practices are shared; (4) ensuring business unit engagement, not compliance; (5) tracking and reporting business unit results to the corporate champion; and (6) providing integration for cross-business unit processes.

The value that champions can bring to an EHR implementation is often overlooked. However, the role is of such importance that Miller, Sim, and Newman, in their report entitled, "Electronic Medical Records: Lessons from Small Physician Practices" stated, "Identify an EMR champion—or don't implement" (2003, p. 7). Their advice is equally appropriate in any size implementation. A champion's efforts greatly impact in multiple implementations, not only in leading the project forward, but in providing support to those colleagues who may not be so enthusiastic about the implementation. Effective champions—generally physicians—who are valued and respected as leaders, and who are perceived to be "one of us" by their peers, contribute significantly to a successful EHR implementation.

Belts

The final positions that George describes are called belts. The four levels of belts (Master Black, Black, Green, and White) are thoroughly trained individuals who have a process view of the organization in addition to application expertise. Each belt level has a slightly different responsibility.

Master Black Belt.   These individuals provide internal expert consultation to black belts and their teams. They must be skilled leaders and expert resources. Master Black Belts provide the conduit to get best practices communicated with unit champions and the rest of the organization. Because most organizations do not have enough employees that hold these skills at the beginning of an EHR venture, it is common to use the experience of external consultants who bring knowledge from prior implementations. Eventually, the consultants will turn over their responsibilities to internal resources.

Black Belt.   Black Belts are responsible for delivering project value and benefits. They work with the line manager and unit champions, identify best practices, and act as mentors. They must be extensively trained in the technology. Some organizations refer to this role as a "Super User" or "Site Specialist." In some cases, the Super Users may become vendor certified in an application, and they might be part of a training team. The Black Belt must be enthusiastic about the implementation and have strong technology skills. It is ideal to identify clinicians and other health care providers as Super Users, because they utilize the technology in their everyday duties, understand the workflow of a unit, and can act as resources to colleagues.

Green Belt.   These individuals are team members who receive significant training and possess knowledge that is important to the project's success. Clinicians and members of the health care team who use the EHR on a daily basis fit this role.

White Belt.   These individuals have some understanding of the EHR, but may use only pieces of the application in their daily duties. Examples include medical records or laboratory staff, who need to access the EHR for "view only" purposes or to perform minimal data entry.

In summary, there are numerous roles and responsibilities in an EHR implementation. Identifying these roles and assigning team members to them early in the project will contribute significantly to a successful outcome.

Training

Training is often placed near the bottom of an implementation project plan; however, it deserves a prominent place prior to, during, and long after an EHR implementation. In fact, training never stops. It is not a one-time endeavor. When

Amatayakul refers to training, her advice is to "train, train, and train" (p. 19). Unfortunately, training rarely gets the attention that it deserves. Some of the more common reasons are:

1. Health care training is expensive. Clinicians are generally among the higher-paid members in an organization and, when they are released from patient care responsibilities to attend training, replacements may have to be hired to cover for them. Clinicians also use a greater proportion of the EHR functionality, so their training times are longer than other employee groups. It is common to require 20 or more hours of training during an implementation when integrating a full-featured EHR.

2. The amount of training required to achieve competency is often underestimated. Vendors frequently advertise their systems as easy to learn; however, these claims may not be reflected in the classroom. Training is more than knowing what button to click; it involves re-training to master new ways of performing numerous workflows.

3. Organizations focus their spending on the technology rather than on human resources. By the time training begins in some organizations, expenditures may already be well beyond anticipated costs, and the training budget is an easy target. Administrators may base the number of hours they will fund based upon financial constraints rather than the amount of time it takes clinicians to meet learning objectives.

The organization that skimps on training prior to an implementation will end up paying for it in other ways that may not be directly attributed in a training department's budget. If learners are not able to reach competency prior to a go-live, they will generally require reduced schedules and patient loads for longer periods of time, and they will require more intensive 1:1 on-site post-implementation support. Although reduced schedules and on-site support are part of any implementation, these are very expensive support methods that, with proper planning and sufficient learner training opportunities, can be significantly reduced.

Technology-Based Training

Classroom-based, instructor-led training is the traditional approach for learning EHRs. Classroom instruction, although effective, can often be supplemented and, in some instances, replaced by technology-assisted instruction such as Web-based training (WBT). WBT has significant advantages in comparison to classroom-based training (Ellis, Wagner, & Longmire, 1999):

- Addresses learning at the individual level
- Can be designed for use anytime and anywhere

- Can be designed to be learner-driven at a pace that corresponds to an individual's learning style
- Can be used at the trainee's job site, as time is available
- Does not require additional physical space
- Connects learners in diverse locations
- Enables immediate implementation of new learning
- Facilitates seamless connection between training and performance support

Leading large, multi-facility, enterprise-wide WBT training initiatives in which clinicians were able to quickly learn basic EHR functionality is indeed possible, but requires customized training to meet the needs of various role-based groups. In addition, by using cutting-edge technologies, the course developers were able to assemble course content with such precision that a particular lesson could include, or exclude as needed, content at the task level. Because each task represented approximately 1.5 minutes of content, learners were offered only content that was relevant for their work. The WBT was supplemented by instructor-led training where clinicians could work in a simulated environment, learn more about incorporating the EHR into their daily workflow, and integrate what they learned. Although expensive to develop, WBT should be considered as a training adjunct whenever large numbers of people with varying roles require training.

It is important for learners to practice in a simulated EHR environment before working in a "live" system, one that exactly parallels the job's data flow. This provides an opportunity for trial and error, time to experiment with personalizing areas of the system if functionality permits, and to develop speed in using the application. It also provides the clinician with an opportunity to see how end-to-end processes are handled in the system. Thus, the creation and maintenance of a training environment with realistic-appearing clinical data is a valuable tool in implementing an EHR.

DATA INFRASTRUCTURE

Data are a key component that bring value to EHRs and provide EBP support. Although data are present in every organization, the difference between data in health care organizations is that health care data are a greater challenge to capture, store, and process because of their textual and contextual nature (Amatayakul). Thus, the design of the data infrastructure, including the architecture, vocabulary, and quality contribute to the value of the EHR.

Humans have the ability to combine data collected by reading and through their senses, and to enhance that data with their experience. This results in knowledge. Computers, although able to process data rapidly and tirelessly, cannot create knowledge without humans programming them with complex structures that attempt to simulate human thinking. Computers with their sources of data, information, and knowledge can be very useful to clinicians when they need to rapidly collect and process numerous facts and quickly make decisions (Amatayakul).

EHR Data Types

An EHR will contain multiple data formats because clinical data come in many different forms. Kohn, in Amatayakul's book (2004) defines seven different formats:

1. Document Image Data. Handwritten notes and drawings; signed patient consent forms.
2. Discrete, Structured Data. Laboratory orders and results, medication orders and MARS, online charting and documentation, and master person index and registration data.
3. Diagnostic Image Data. Computed tomography (CT), magnetic resonance (MR), digital X-rays, nuclear medicine, and pathology/histology images.
4. Vector Graphic Data. Electrocardiogram (EKG), electroencephalogram (EEG), and fetal signal tracings.
5. Audio Data. Heart sounds and voice annotation.
6. Video Data. Ultrasound and cardiac catheterization examinations.
7. Unstructured Text Data. Transcribed radiology and pathology reports, and itemized bills.

Kohn suggested that Document Image Data, and Discrete Structured Data are the major data types, with each comprising 25% of the total content.

Vocabulary and Classifications

It is important to develop and adopt vocabulary, classification standards, and codes to reduce inconsistency and to ensure understanding among health care providers. Although entire chapters could be devoted to these topics, these concepts are briefly covered because it is helpful for the clinician to understand how these are interrelated and support EBP.

It is important to carefully select and apply vocabulary standards for the EHR to be able to properly extract meaning. In some cases, terminology may be prescribed. As an example, the American Medical Association's Common Procedural Terminology is a set of terms used for professional billing. An EHR is also dependent upon a nomenclature that is a defined naming system. The Systematized Nomenclature of Medicine (SNOMED) is health care's most widely recognized nomenclature and is developed and managed by the College of American Pathologists. SNOMED Clinical Terms (SNOMED CT®), the most current version, provides a set of concepts and relationships that provide a common reference point for comparison and aggregation of health care process data (Amatayakul). SNOMED CT® also contains nursing terminologies such as: (1) Nursing Diagnoses: Definitions and Classification; (2) Nursing Interventions Classifications; (3) Nursing Outcomes Classification; (4) Perioperative Nursing Data Set; and (5) the Omaha System.

A classification system groups terms of similar meaning. The most widely recognized medical classification system is the International Classification of Diseases. Amatayakul (2004) suggests that a classification system alone is inadequate for an EHR where clinical decision support rests on very specific data. However, she posited that the systems should be coordinated and stated that the National Library of Medicine does map ICD-9-CM and other classification systems to SNOMED.

Data Structures

Data structure refers to the specific way each data element is used in an information system. By controlling vocabulary, standardizing terminology, and classifications, data can more easily be captured, managed, and retrieved.

In April 2004, President George W. Bush issued Executive Order 13335, calling for the widespread adoption of interoperable EHRs within 10 years. To meet this goal, standardization of data structure and data architecture is becoming increasingly important. Standardization supports the interoperability of health information across health care environments. This will enable consumers to have their medical information move seamlessly with them when they change clinicians or geographic locations. Without an interoperable infrastructure to allow for the secure movement of health information, the adoption and use of EHRs will not achieve their full benefits (Thompson & Brailer).

THE FUTURE

The innovation and development of new technologies, and the diffusion of those technologies into health care environments, will most certainly contribute to the ability of clinicians to access clinical data and apply EBP. Wireless and mobile technologies such as Tablet PCs, Personal Digital Assistants, and smart cell phone technologies will contribute to patient health data and CDSS access at the point of care.

As stated earlier, technology is the bridge to integrating EBP into patient care.

REFERENCES

The American Heritage Dictionary. (2001). New York: Dell Publishing.

Amatayakul, M. K. (2004). *Electronic Health Records: A Practical Guide for Professionals and Organizations.* Chicago: American Health Information Management Association.

Beck, E. (2004). Analysis: Meeting the E-Record Challenge. Available at http://www.upi.com/view/cfm?StoryID=20040721-121144-4038r. Retrieved February 2005.

Brailer, D. J., & Terasawa, E. L. (2003). *Use and Adoption of Computer-Based Patient Records.* Oakland, CA: California HealthCare Foundation.

Briggs, B. (2004). Clinical systems move to the head of the I.T. Class. *Health Data Management.* Stamford, CT: The Thompson Corporation and Health Data Management.

Covell, D., Uman, G., & Manning, P. (1985). Information needs in office practice: Are they being met? *Annals of Internal Medicine, 103*(4), 596–599.

D'Alessandro, D. M., Kreiter, C. D., & Peterson, M. W. (2004). An evaluation of information-seeking behaviors of general pediatricians. *Pediatrics, 113*(1), 64–69.

Doncaster, B., & Hunter Harvey, S. (2003). A macro-analytic perspective on e-learning: The context. In R. C. Geibert & S. Hunter Harvey (Eds.), *Web-Wise Learning: Wisdom from the Field.* Philadelphia: Xlibris Corporation, Inc.

Ellis, A. L., Wagner, E. D., & Longmire, W. R. (1999). *Managing Web-Based Training.* Alexandria, VA: American Society for Training & Development.

Ely, J. W., Osheroff, J. A., Ebell, M. H., Chambliss, M. L., Vinson, D. C., & Stevermer, J. J., et al. (2002). Obstacles to answering doctors' questions about patient care with evidence: Qualitative study. *British Medical Journal, 324*(7339), 710–716.

Fact Sheet: Bibliographic Services Division. (2003). Available at http://www.nlm.nih.gov/pubs/factsheets/bsd.html. Retrieved February 2005.

Fox, S., & Fallows, D. (2003). Health searches and email have become more commonplace, but there is room for improvement in searches and overall internet access. Available at http://www.pewinternet.org/pdfs/PIP_Health_Report_July_2003.pdf. Retrieved February 2005.

George, M. L. (2002). *Lean Six Sigma: Combining Six Sigma Quality with Lean Speed.* New York: McGraw-Hill.

Greenspan, R. (2004). Active internet users by country, June 2004. Available at http://www.clickz.com/stats/big_picture/geographics/article.php/3386051. Retrieved February 2005.

HealthGrades. (2004). In-hospital deaths from medical errors at 195,000 per year, Healthgrades' study finds. Available at http://www.healthgrades.com/AboutUs/index.cfm?fuseaction=mod&modtype=content&modact=Media_PressRelease_Detail&&press_id=135. Retrieved February 2005.

HHS Fact Sheet—HIT Report at-a-Glance. (2004). Available at http://www.hhs.gov/news/press/2004pres/20040721.html. Retrieved February 2005.

Hunter Harvey, S., & Geibert, R. (2003). An organizational approach: Web development from a systems perspective. In R. Geibert and S. Hunter Harvey (Eds.), *Web-Wise Learning: Wisdom from the Field.* Philadelphia: XLibris Corporation; pp. 19–22.

Johnston, M. E., Langton, K. B., Haynes, B., & Mathieu, A. (1994). Effects of computer-based clinical decision support systems on clinician performance and patient outcome. *Annals of Internal Medicine, 120*(2), 135–142.

Kaiser Permanente. (1999). *Evidence-Based Medicine.* Oakland, CA: Kaiser Permanente.

McGlynn, E., Asch, S., Adams, J., Keesey, J., Hicks, J., DeCristofaro, A., et al. (2003). The quality of health care delivered to adults in the United States. *The New England Journal of Medicine, 348*(26), 2635–2645.

Medical Records Institute's Sixth Annual Survey of Electronic Health Record Trends and Usage for 2004. Available at http://www.medrecinst.com/pages/latestNews.asp?id=115. Retrieved February 2005.

Miller, R. H., Sim, I., & Newman, J. (2003). Electronic medical records: Lessons from small physician practices. Available at http://www.chcf.org/documents/ihealth/EMRLessonsSmallPhysician Practices.pdf. Retrieved 9/4/04.

Osheroff, J. A., Forsythe, D. E., Buchanan, B. G., Bankowitz, R. A., Blumenfeld, B. H., & Miller, R. A. (1991). Physician's information needs: Analysis of questions posed during clinical teaching. *Annals of Internal Medicine, 114*, 576–581.

Rae, S., & O'Driscoll, T. (2004). Contextualized learning: Empowering education. In *Chief Learning Officer*. Oakland, CA: MediaTec Publishing, Inc.

Randolph, A., Haynes, R. B., Wyatt, J., Cook, D., & Guyatt, G. (2001). How to use an article evaluating the clinical impact of a computer-based clinical decision support system. Available at http://www.cche.net/usersguides/computer.asp. Retrieved February 2005.

Rosenberg, M. J. (2001). *E-Learning: Strategies for Delivering Knowledge in the Digital Age*. New York: McGraw-Hill.

Sackett, D., Rosenberg, W. M., Gray, J. M., Haynes, B., & Richardson, W. S. (1996). Evidence-based medicine: What it is and what it isn't. *British Medical Journal, 312*(7023), 71–72.

Thompson, T. G., & Brailer, D. J. (2004). The decade of health information technology: Delivering consumer-centric and information-rich health care: Framework for strategic action. Washington, DC: Department of Health & Human Services.

Underwood, A. (2004, August 2). Hospital horrors. *Newsweek, CXLIV*, 12.

CHAPTER 7

Managing Variance Through an Evidence-Based Framework for Safe and Reliable Health Care

Kathy A. Scott

Health care in the United States is dependent on good people (from novice to expert) doing the right things (often despite evidence) at the right time (despite numerous interruptions and distractions). While the United States has the capacity to produce the greatest health care in the world, research clearly indicates that the health care industry has failed to do so with shocking regularity (Becher & Chassin, 2001). Health care errors represent the seventh leading cause of death in this country (Grube, 2001), resulting in 44,000 to 98,000 deaths per year, and costing the nation approximately $376 billion annually (Institute of Medicine (IOM), 1999). Misdiagnoses of patients experiencing a myocardial infarction in the emergency department are estimated at 20,000 to 80,000 per million (Merry & Brown, 2002). The estimated cost of nonfatal medical errors is $17 to 19 billion each year (Rovner, 2000), an estimated cost of $2,500–$3,500 per hospital bed/year for medication errors alone (Coile, 2001). Research also indicates that between 2.9% and 3.7% of all hospital admissions result in an injury from mismanagement (Benjamin, 2000), and 5.75% of hospitalized patients experience preventable adverse events (that is, an injury judged to be the result of an error or system design flaw) within two weeks following discharge (Forster, Murff, Peterson, Gandhi, & Bates, 2003).

High-reliability organizations (HROs) are complex systems that have a very different view of the organization and how it works, a view that is far removed from the traditional health care paradigm. HRO members collectively understand that uncertainty is irreducible, sources of harm are limitless, and that human factors have a significant effect on outcomes. They share a common set of attributes and practices that make them much more safe and reliable than the rest (Becher & Chassin, 2001; Weick & Sutcliffe, 2001).

This chapter explores and integrates the essence of evidence-based practice—best research, clinical expertise, and patient-focused values—and relates them to a high-reliability framework for managing process and outcome variability for safe patient care. Through strategies derived from an evidence-based high-reliability framework, leaders are able to make better-informed decisions and effectively manage the organization in ways that decrease errors, promote employee retention, and improve patient outcomes.

RELIABILITY DEFINED

Reliability is the extent to which a system yields the same results on repeated trials. A highly reliable system is one that is error-tolerant; it has consistent and positive results. A reliable health care system is not a product of everyone's hard work, best efforts, or good intentions. Rather, it is designed to ensure that every patient receives evidence-based and effective care every time, regardless of the time of day, day of the week, or participants' gender, expertise, ethnicity, or socio-economic status.

Highly reliable practices and organizations are the result of individuals, teams, and systems that together: (1) mitigate the effects of harmful variation/error; (2) prevent harm caused by variation/error; and/or (3) prevent the variation/error from happening in the first place. A framework is needed to view organizations in new ways that will help leaders actively prevent and/or manage the risks of active and latent failures at all levels of the organization.

HIGH-RISK AND COMPLEX HEALTH CARE SYSTEMS

Health care organizations have the defining characteristics of high risk and complexity. The more complex the system, the more likely it is that a random mix of events will combine to produce a mishap. Within a larger frame of reference, factors that produce small and subtle effects can have very large consequences. Seven characteristics of complex systems are identified from the literature, as presented in Table 7.1, which make them highly accident/failure-prone regardless of the intent of the leaders or members/actors.

Two complex system characteristics are identified by Perrow (1984), a researcher of accidents in high-risk industries, as being highly accident prone regardless of the intent of their leaders or members:

- Interactive complexity: A measure of the way in which parts are connected and interact. According to Perrow, complex interactions are unplanned, unexpected, and unfamiliar sequences that are either not visible or not immediately comprehensible.

Table 7.1   Seven Characteristics of Complex Systems That Lead to Breakdown and Failure

1. Interactive complexity
2. Tight coupling
3. Conflicting goals
4. Intransparence
5. Fluid participation
6. Dynamic with complex delays
7. Ignorance and mistaken assumptions

- Tight coupling: Planned and unplanned interactions that occur quickly when delays in the process are not possible. There is little slack in the system and precision must be there the first time or not at all.

March, Cohen, and Olsen defined the presence of three general characteristics in complex organizations (Sagan, 1993) that are also reflective of health care organizations.

- Conflicting goals: There are inconsistent, conflicting, and differing goals at many different levels of the organization.
- Intransparence: Many aspects of the organization are not visible or are unclear. Organizational processes and influences are not well understood by the actors, planners, and decision-makers, who often do not have direct access to information about the situation they are addressing.
- Fluid participation: The organizational participants are coming and going with some paying attention and some not. Members of the decision-making groups are often uninformed, biased, or even uninterested actors.

Dietrich Dörner (1996), an internationally respected figure in the field of cognitive behavior and human error, identified the three characteristics above as well as two additional properties of complex systems that lead to breakdown and failure:

- Dynamic with complex delays: The system is always moving and changing on its own whether the actors take it into account or not. Decisions have to be made before complete information is available, and it is difficult to determine where the whole system is heading over time. There are many unrecognized system delays and side effects.

* Ignorance and mistaken assumptions: The organizational actors rely on and apply their past reality model (implicit and explicit) to situations whether they have been effective or not in the past.

Health care organizations are high risk in that error, failure, and breakdown can lead to loss of life or body function. Health care organizations exhibit the seven evidence-based characteristics of complex systems. They are opaque, with many subsystems of specialists and services dependent on each other for information. These subsystems are often not well understood by planners, leaders, or patient-care providers. Health care systems are tightly coupled, requiring rapid decisions during unexpected situations where individuals and groups are unstable, personally threatened, or threatening to others.

Health care systems have many parts that are interdependent in an environment where planned and unplanned interactions occur quickly and have serious consequences. In the operating room, for example, coronary bypass surgery requires the interaction of many team members with a variety of skill levels, communication styles, abilities, high-tech equipment, coordination of processes, and timely precision with no second chances for many actions that impact the surgical procedure and experience. Imagine the immediate outcome of a distracted perfusion technician who forgets to prime the coronary artery tubing with saline prior to starting the case. The result would be a cardiac arrest from an air embolus within seconds. Likewise, even a short delay in the circulating RN's double check of the patient's surgical consent form at the time of surgery could result in the performance of the wrong surgical procedure for a patient due to tight coupling from the time in the operating room to the time of incision.

From a more administrative perspective, leadership decisions such as those related to human resource management, supply contracts and purchases, and productivity benchmarks, exert a tremendous influence on organizational reliability and safety as well. A decision in the boardroom to purchase an inferior infusion pump can result in errors by the end-user that are not understood, immediately visible, or comprehensible. Because of the complexity of the system, the decision-maker may never have any understanding of his or her contribution to the harm that occurs.

Clinically, ignorance and mistaken hypotheses are evident as traditional medical and clinical practices continue even after research clearly indicates a better way to improve outcomes. Practitioners are overloaded and desire to practice autonomously, often performing in ways that are most expedient and comfortable for them. Health care leaders have been reluctant to standardize care and practice based on the evidence because of political pressures and mistaken assumptions, such as the notion that diagnosis and treatment of disease require very specialized and individualized knowledge and experience.

Conflicting goals, ambiguous preferences, and conflicting interests often coexist in a state of uneasy tension in health care organizations. Leaders and other employees often take the easier path of generalization and political ease, paying only arbitrary attention to the details of the trade-offs, and hope for the best. A study (Pronovost, Angus, Dorman, Robinson, Dremsizov, & Young, 2002) of intensive care units (ICUs) demonstrates this point of conflicting goals in health care organizations. When patients were managed or co-managed by physician intensivists, there were associated reductions in hospital mortality (30%) and ICU mortality (40%). These data suggest that more than 160,000 of the deaths that occur in the U.S. ICUs annually could be avoided. Yet, it is estimated that only 10% of ICUs in the United States have this type of staffing (Pronovost et al.). This evidence-based practice has become well known in the health care industry through The Leapfrog Group, a consortium of over 160 companies and organizations (health care consumers) with a mission to improve the quality and affordability of health care in the United States. However, political and professional interests, such as physicians not wanting to relinquish any of their patient care privileges, control, or revenue in the ICU setting to the Intensivist, are often placed ahead of the patients' interests, resulting in higher mortality rates and injuries from errors.

There is a dual-minded organizational structure in health care organizations that differs substantially from that of other industries and contributes to its complexity. The chief executive officer (CEO) receives delegated authority from the board and is responsible for managing the organization with the senior management team. The medical staff constitutes a separate organizational structure parallel to the administrative structure. The medical staffs are generally not paid employees of the hospital, yet they play a significant role in its success (Shi & Singh, 2001). Often the two groups have different agendas, expectations, goals, and views of situations with numerous competing interests and conflicts. The result is similar to a body with two heads, with each head having a different view of the world. Competing interests, hierarchical views, conflicts, and cultures that promote competition and avoidance are often the result. This is a recipe for complexity and failure.

Conflicting and differing goals are evident within the nursing world as well, creating tension from two competing goods. Examples are the tension between standardization and individualized care; cost containment and specialized care; and care for the individual and care for the collective. Day-to-day decisions around diverting patients to other hospitals versus holding or admitting when nurses believe their ability to provide safe patient care may be jeopardized is commonly found across the United States and exemplifies the tension from two competing goals.

Fluid participation is evident in health care organizations. Health care organizations have multiple member groups with voluntary turnover rates of one-fifth to one-quarter annually as well as physician-actors who have a separate leadership structure, great independence in their practice, and many conflicts-of-interest with the health care organization in which they provide services. Other contributors to fluid participation include 24/7 work schedules, and unexpected patient care situations that require immediate attention and divert the actors' time and ability to participate in nonpatient care activities.

Through recognition of the seven characteristics present in nonrational, high-risk, and complex health care organizations (interactive complexity, tight coupling, conflicting goals, intransparence, fluid participation, dynamic with complex delays, and ignorance and mistaken assumptions), new approaches will evolve that encourage a more realistic look at the antecedents and root causes of variance, practice breakdown, and organizational failures. This next section identifies many of the human tendencies when problem solving in complex situations that lead to variance, failures, and breakdown.

LEADERSHIP AND PROBLEM-SOLVING PITFALLS IN COMPLEX SYSTEMS

Dietrich Dörner, a researcher in the field of cognitive psychology, has extensively studied the nature of human thinking when dealing with complex problems. Using computer simulations at the University of Bambuerg, Dörner mapped out the strengths and weaknesses of human cognition when confronted with complex problem-solving environments. He identified "habits of thought that set failure in motion from the beginning" (1987, p. 11). Through the development of simulated complex situations for interactive problem-solving that did not require any particular technical expertise, Dörner was able to observe and record the background of planning, decision-making, and evaluation processes that were usually hidden. Dörner's research, combined with the findings of several other scholars, revealed six human tendencies when problem solving in complex situations. These tendencies are outlined in Table 7.2.

Difficulty Understanding Delays

The primary mistakes or errors made by almost all subjects during the simulated scenarios were insufficient consideration of processes in time with the tendency to think in terms of isolated cause-and-effect relationships. Each of these mistakes was related to the phenomenon of delays from the time of one's

Table 7.2   Human Tendencies When Problem Solving in Complex Systems

1. Difficulty understanding the consequences of delays with isolated cause-and-effect thinking
2. Deterioration of planful thinking and disconfirming evidence
3. Simplify and economize
4. Preserve an optimistic view of oneself
5. Focus on the symptoms versus the fundamental issues
6. Neglect to reflect on the consequences of past decisions

action to the consequences. Under time pressure, the participants had a tendency to apply overdoses of established measures (Dörner, 1996).

Deterioration of Planful Thinking

With repetitive failures, all participants in Dörner's study (1996) demonstrated a deterioration of "planful thinking." This was defined as a marked increase in willingness to bend the rules as failures repeated; reductive hypotheses, attributing all phenomena to a single cause; and confirmation biases that became more marked, with participants looking for evidence that confirmed their thinking rather than disconfirmed (Reason, 1990).

In addition to difficulty with the phenomenon of delays (from the time of one's action to the consequences) and deterioration of planful thinking, four human failings were evident in the research of problem-solving tendencies in complex situations. They are the tendency to simplify and economize; preserve an optimistic view of oneself; focus on the symptoms versus the fundamental issues; and neglect to reflect on the consequences of their past decisions.

Tendency to Simplify

The tendency to economize or simplify when planning by not taking side effects and long-term repercussions into account is when all effort goes toward treating the symptom(s) and not toward solving the underlying problem, because it is difficult and time consuming to obtain the knowledge about all the possible interactions with a particular system that led to the underlying problem (Weick & Sutcliffe, 2001). Humans prefer to develop and/or maintain a hypothesis, ignoring information that does not conform to it, and responding to the similarities (Dörner, 1996; Reason, 1990). Truth is commonly identified with comprehensibility and simplicity. What one does not understand is rejected as false (Gharajedaghi, 1999).

Delusional Optimism

A second reason for poor decision-making in complex situations is the tendency to preserve an optimistic view about one's abilities and accomplishments. Lovallo and Dahneman (2003), a business scholar and psychologist, respectively, referred to this tendency of executives as "delusional optimism." Research into human cognition has traced being overly optimistic to many sources, with one of the most powerful being the tendency of individuals to exaggerate their own talents, believing they are above average in their endowment. The inclination to exaggerate one's talents is amplified by the tendency to misperceive the causes of, and degree of control over, certain events. Executives, especially, seem to be highly susceptible to these biases (Lovallo and Dahneman).

Dörner's research (1996) identified the tendency to preserve a positive view of oneself as an attribution failure that lay outside the realm of cognitive processes. These preservation acts contributed significantly to shaping the direction and course of the participants' thought processes. Argyris' research (1991) observed that many professionals have difficulty learning from their errors because they so rarely experience them. He continued with the observation that when professionals commit errors, they become defensive, screen out criticism, and push the blame on others. It was his view that their ability to learn shuts down precisely at the moment they need it the most. This act of self-protection is essential—to a point—to maintain a minimum capacity to act (Dörner) but becomes a barrier without a healthy dose of realism (Lovallo & Dahneman, 2003).

Symptom Thinking versus System Thinking

The third human tendency when dealing with complex situations is to focus on the wrong problems and goals, neglecting the fundamental issues and their long-term considerations and consequences. This so-called "repair-service behavior" occurs when partial or interim goals capture the participant's attention and displace the primary goals (Dörner, 1996). Often the tasks that become the focus are those that the individual feels competent doing and challenged by, with the reward of gratification of some success. The partial goals are often in contradictory relationships to the primary goal, which are not always evident. This leads to actions that inevitably replace one problem with another and a resulting vicious cycle.

Neglect to Reflect

Studies indicate that neither intelligence nor specialized experience or motivation differentiate the high performers from the low performers (Dörner, 1996; Goleman, 1998; Senge, 1990). The difference is in the knowledge that individuals have about the use of their intellectual capabilities and skills. Successful individuals are those who are capable of approaching problems in a variety of ways, learning as they go along.

Those who reflect on their own thinking and feeling and learn from their experiences demonstrate better problem-solving abilities. They are able to "make meaning" out of the experience they and others have in the world (Dixon, 1999) through recognizing their own underlying decision-making tendencies, emotional habits, assumptions, and unexpected side effects of earlier actions. This ability to make meaning requires an individual to pause and consider that there are relationships in the world that one cannot readily see, and to consider that one creates the world in which he or she lives through preferences of interpreting the world. Reflection with courage enhances an individual's ability to feel the dissonance that is experienced when one denies the validity of a situation, which can be used to then reconstruct new understanding of it.

LEADERSHIP'S VIEW: EFFECT ON RELIABILITY

A leader's view of the organization and how it works has a profound impact on the organization's reliability—or ability to yield the same results on repeated trials. Therefore, a precursor to creating more highly reliable organizations is a "highly reliable" view of health care organizations. There is a successive shift in the understanding of the nature of organizations and how they work across the country. However, the health care industry is lagging in this understanding, which results in decision-making that detracts from its viability and reliability. This next section describes three views of organizational leaders that impact outcome variance and reliability: a biological view, multi-minded view, and high-reliability view.

Biological ("Uni-minded") View of Organizations

The biological (or "uni-minded") view is the dominant perspective found in many organizations today. This view emerged mainly in Germany and Britain and then spread to the United States. An organization is considered a uni-minded living system, similar to the traditional Western view of the human body, with a purpose of its own. That purpose is survival and comes from the inherent vulnerability and unstable structure of open systems. To survive, according to conventional wisdom, biological beings have to grow. To grow, humans exploit their environment to achieve a positive metabolism. In organizational language, this means that growth is the measure of success, and profit is the measure to achieve it (Gharajedaghi, 1999). This is very similar to a "marketplace" view where medical and health care institutions sell the services as commodities in the marketplace with a major goal of cost containment for survival purposes.

A "Multi-Minded" Organizational View:
A Precursor to High-Reliability

A precursor to an HRO is a socio-cultural ("multi-minded") view of organizations, or one which considers the organization a voluntary association of purposeful members who themselves manifest a choice of "both ends and means" (Gharajedaghi, 1999). This is a fundamentally different view of organizations than the biological model; it is purposeful because of its purposeful members who manifest choice. The members of a socio-cultural organization are held together by one or more common objectives and collectively acceptable ways of pursuing them. The members share values that are embedded in their culture, and the culture is the cement that integrates the parts into a cohesive whole (Senge, 1990). Because the parts do have something to say about the organization of the whole, consensus is essential to the alignment of a socio-cultural system (Gharajedaghi).

A High-Reliability View of Organizations

HROs are high-risk systems that continuously operate under trying conditions and have fewer than their fair share of accidents. HROs share two essential characteristics: (1) they constantly confront the unexpected, and (2) they operate with remarkable consistency and effectiveness (Weick & Sutcliffe, 2001). HROs do not claim to be immune to catastrophes. Rather, they are distinguished by cultures of safety that include a collective view that recognizes their vulnerability to failure with a willingness to learn from trial-and-error through devotion of time, attention, and effort to avoiding and/or minimizing variation and error. A common characteristic in HROs is that safety behaviors are collectively encouraged rather than discouraged (Klein, Bigley, & Roberts, 1995; Reason, 2000; Weick & Sutcliffe). A high-reliability view of organization perceives the members as the frontline of protection against error and failure who are supported by systems that are designed for failure prevention. HROs understand that uncertainty is irreducible and sources of harm are limitless. Therefore, they anticipate the worst and equip themselves to deal with the unexpected at all levels of the organization.

CULTURES OF DEVIANCE

Culture is "the set of shared attitudes, values, goals, and practices that characterize a company or corporation" (*Merriam-Webster*, 2002). An organization's culture is often referred to as "the way things happen around here" or "the hidden rules that rule behavior." Within most health care organizations, there are social hierarchies or social stratifications that have a profound impact upon the relationships, communication practices, management of conflict, expectations for collaboration, displays of emotion, and patient care practices (Malloch & Porter-O'Grady, 2005).

Health care organizations, rather than having cultures that promote safety, are noted for having cultures of blame, which create incentives that have detrimental effects on safety (Becher & Chassin, 2001). A disaster from the nuclear industry promotes understanding of the negative effects of some cultures with parallels to health care. In the Chernobyl disaster of 1986, a Ukrainian atomic-energy plant in Chernobyl, USSR exploded, destroying its concrete roof that weighed thousands of tons, and polluting the surrounding territory and all of Europe with radioactive particles. A key contributor to the event was the frequent violation of safety rules by the Chernobyl engineers (Dörner, 1996), or "normalization of deviance" (Fountain, 1999). Breaking safety rules had become the norm at that plant, continuously reinforced by no immediate negative consequences as well as the positive consequences of acting more freely by getting rid of the encumbrances that rules imposed.

Health care cultures are rich with deviances that have become normalized. The medical profession, for example, has both formal and informal peer-review processes that often grant forgiveness, deny, silence, discount, and/or cover up errors (Smith & Forster, 2000). The nursing profession often ignores poor clinical judgment and interpersonal skills of avoidance or aggression until a major event occurs. This nursing tendency to ignore is often related to lack of resources (nurses and/or managers), of standards for accountability, and skills to hold each other accountable.

The IOM's report on *Keeping Patients Safe* (IOM, 2004) identifies three organizational elements that are critical for managing variation and promoting an effective safety culture: environmental structures and processes within the organization; the attitudes and perceptions of the workers; and the safety-related behaviors of individuals. Each element is addressed through a high-reliability framework in the following section.

MANAGING VARIANCE THROUGH A HIGH-RELIABILITY FRAMEWORK

HROs share a common set of ideas and practices that could serve as a framework for health care organizations. More specifically, six evidence-based characteristics of HROs that are applicable to health care leaders and organizations today are learning from feedback, effective teamwork, anticipating the unexpected, deferring to expertise, being extra-sensitive to operations, and reluctance to simplify. The acronym *LEADER*, as shown in Table 7.3, emphasizes the critical importance of purposeful and relentless leadership in creating HROs that minimize variation and promote positive outcomes. This work is a fundamental change in thinking, rather than an incremental process of change. In this perspective, patient care breakdown and errors are seen primarily as a result of practitioners becoming overwhelmed by unsafe conditions rather than as the fault of a single individual who failed. This view, however, is balanced by a "fair

Table 7.3   Six Attributes of High-Reliability Organizations for Health Care Leaders

L	Learn from feedback
E	Effective teamwork
A	Anticipate the unexpected
D	Defer to expertise
E	Extra-sensitive to operations
R	Reluctance to simplify

Source: Reprinted with permission from the unpublished dissertation Errors and Failures in Complex Health-care Systems: Individual, Team, System, and Cultural Contributors, by K. A. Scott, 2004.

and just culture," which seeks to compensate for human error rather than blame, and requires accountability for reporting and learning, rather than perfection. It is balanced by sanctions for the few who knowingly violate the rules and disrupt the workplace.

Learn from Feedback

A paradox of organizational learning is that organizations can learn only through their individual members, yet organizations create systemic constraints that prevent their individual members from learning (Dixon, 1999). Some familiar organizational practices that limit learning are transferring poor performing employees from one department to another rather than out the door; implementing programs that implementers know will not solve the problem due to political or other pressures, softening (or neutralizing) bad news until it is not understood, concealing an unattractive program within an attractive one, and getting the agreement of principal players before a meeting while acting in the meeting as though no such agreement has been reached. Defensive routines occur from these accepted and often tacit practices that result in continued poor performance, unaddressed problems, and lack of learning (Dixon).

Sagan's research (1993) identified strong disincentives for exposing the serious failures that occurred at the National Aeronautics and Space Administration, which are applicable to the health care industry. These disincentives influenced the reporting of near-misses by members, the beliefs of the members related to what was acceptable to report and record, and the public interpretation of events by senior leaders. Two sets of records (one for insiders and one for outsiders) were created and careful instructions given to the actors about what conversations could occur where and when. These activities veiled the actor's internal perceptions, the recording and use of history, and the ability to learn from past mistakes. In fact, research demonstrated that organizations do turn the experience of failure into a memory of success, which further obstructs the organization's ability to learn from their failures.

Dörner's study (1996) identified the tendency of poor performers to act hastily and with reluctance to gather information when in complex situations. Organizations often perpetuate this tendency toward activity (acting eagerly) through rewarding swift action as if it were competence and discouraging inaction such as dialogue and reflection. Organizational psychologist Karl Weick identifies "action, tempered by reflection" as a critical component for organizational success when operating in the strange, chaotic, and unfamiliar (Coutu, 2003).

Another observed phenomenon that prevents learning is observed with "smart" people (such as health care professionals) who rarely experience or are unaware of experiencing failure (Argyris, 1990). When they do commit an error, they become defensive, screen out criticism, and place the blame on others. It is Argyris' view that smart people's ability to learn shuts down just when they need it most.

HROs create cultures and structures that encourage members to report even small and inconsequential lapses swiftly to facilitate a rapid response for learning and correction. HROs learn from their mistakes as a result of an openness to learn and swift processing of data. Case studies demonstrate that people were candid about the events surrounding a failure for a short period of time, and then they got their story straight in ways that justified their actions and protected their reputations (Weick & Sutcliffe, 2001). In a book on military misfortunes, this truth is revealed: "...on the actual day of battle naked truths may be picked up for the asking. But by the following morning they have already begun to get into their uniforms" (Cohen & Gooch, 1990, p. 44). Determining the root causes of errors and poor performance and identifying high-leverage interventions that will markedly improve performance require swift and nonjudgmental dialogue and action by organizational leadership.

Learning Strategies: Practical Application

Leadership Rounding.   A formula borrowed from ecology states that in order for an organism to survive, its rate of learning must be equal to or greater than the rate of change in its environment. The formula is written $L \geq C$ (Dixon, 1999). One activity to help leaders learn and survive is called "leadership rounding," which is focused on patient and environmental safety. When senior executives (such as the CEO, chief nursing officer, chief medical officer, or chief operating officer) visibly round with staff to explore the variations from safe patient practice, learning is greatly enhanced for all parties, and more effective strategies will result for minimizing variation and improving outcomes. Ten basic steps for effective safety rounds are outlined in Table 7.4 that promote feedback and learning. Leaders—equipped with the belief that vulnerability is inherent in the complex health care system and with a willingness to learn from the people performing the work—must pay particular attention to their words and body language, and avoid reactions and rationalizations for current perceived failures, such as minimizing, denying, blaming, ignoring, or retaliation. The process begins and ends with nonjudgmental dialogue between leadership and staff to create and sustain the trust that is so critical to reporting and managing error/practice breakdown.

Debriefing.   Learning from feedback also requires redesigned structures and/or processes that promote collaborative interaction and objective, forthright communication. The act of debriefing is a constructive discussion of a team's ac-

Table 7.4   Patient Safety Rounds: 10-Step Process

1. Senior leader(s) schedule an appointment to round with staff in their department.
2. Ask staff to identify barriers to their practice that could potentially result in harm.
3. Ask employees to identify recent errors or "near misses."
4. Brainstorm perceived contributors (practitioner competence, team norms, and process design) to errors or "near misses" with employees.
5. Brainstorm actions necessary to prevent events from reoccurring.
6. Communicate next steps in the process.
7. Meet with manager, prioritize issues, and create an action plan around key breakdown areas.
8. Assign responsibility and timelines for actions.
9. Track actions and changes.
10. Provide feedback of actions and outcomes to the original contributors.

tivities quickly after a procedure or event is concluded (Leonard, Graham, & Taggart, 2004). When debriefing expectations and time are built into the day, individual, team, and organizational learning is enhanced. The focus is on promoting situational awareness, reinforcing and rewarding excellence, and identifying opportunities for improvement through dialogue around the following questions: What went well? What would we do differently next time? What made this more difficult? What are the next steps to ensure that performance is improved?

Effective Teamwork

Teams often perform better than individuals. Teamwork is defined as "work done by several associates with each doing a part but all subordinating personal prominence to the efficiency of the whole" (*Merriam-Webster*, 2002). Teamwork matters in health care because most endeavors require groups to work together effectively, with failures often having deadly effects. In the aviation industry, another complex and high-risk industry, more than two-thirds of the air crashes studied involved human error, especially failures in teamwork (Helmreich, 2003). Teams are of primary importance in preventing errors because individuals are imperfect in their skills, motivation, and cognition (Edmondson, 1996); professional training has focused on technical, not interpersonal skills (Helmreich), and organizational systems are inevitably flawed (Edmondson; IOM, 2001; Leape, 1999).

Through the group level phenomenon of synergy, unconscious processes of the group can manifest themselves in the individual member's actions (Alderfer, 1987), creating either positive or negative outcomes collectively, which are quite different from the outcomes that would be obtained by simply adding up the contributions of the individual members working alone (Hackman, 1987; Weick, 1990). Teams in organizations can act as "self-correcting performance units" to counteract the ever-present potential for error (Benner, Hooper-Kyriakidis, & Stannard, 1999) as well as performance units that perpetuate errors and undesired outcomes (Weick). A study (Edmondson, 1996; Foushee, Lauber, Baetge, & Acomb, 1986) of fatigue on flight crew errors in the aviation industry found that crews who were fatigued after working several days together made significantly fewer errors than teams who were well-rested but had not worked together. As expected, the fatigued individuals made more errors than their rested counterparts; but as a team, the group that worked together compensated for each other and overall made fewer errors than the rested team (Edmondson; Sexton, Thomas, & Helmreich, 2000).

Negative effects of the team can occur, however, when members of a work team communicate across tacit boundaries imposed by rank or identity group, inhibiting the transfer of valid data (Argyris, 1985; Edmondson, 1996). Nurses and physicians face group identity boundaries confounded with status differences that can affect within-team communication and patient safety.

Conflict is defined as "a clash or struggle that occurs when a real or perceived threat or difference exists in the desires, thoughts, attitudes, feelings, or behaviors of two or more parties" (Cox, 2003, p. 154). Human needs are at the center of all conflicts. People engage in conflict either because they have needs that they perceive as inconsistent with those of others, or needs that are met by the conflict process itself (Mayer, 2000).

Group conflict refers to both intra- and inter-group conflict. Intra-group conflict is when disagreements or differences exist among members of a particular group or its subgroups, while differences and disagreements between two or more groups or their representatives are referred to as inter-group conflict (Cox, 2003, p. 155). In a survey of nurses employed in 13 different inpatient units, Cox found that intra-group conflict had direct negative effects on work satisfaction and team performance.

Research indicates that trust among members and a sense of group identity are essential conditions to a group's effectiveness (Druskat & Wolff, 2001). Trust is an important ingredient for fully optimizing any system. Without trust, members seek to protect their own immediate interests, to the detriment of the long-term effectiveness and well-being of the entire system (Deming, 1986). Teams and team members have values or principles that guide their behavior often without their awareness. Teams and team members also have daily norms or actions at a more superficial level. When the team members share these values and actions collectively, they are able to develop a sense of group identity.

The social norms of a team may differ significantly from moral norms. Social norms may require that team members support each other by hiding and/or minimizing what goes on within the team. Moral norms, on the other hand, could require blowing the whistle on what is considered unsafe practice, and may be viewed as "tattling" by another team member (Aroskar, 1985). Commitment to the team more than to the patient can result in actions and behaviors that feed the underlying problems in systems and allow them to continue. It can also result in harm to patients. Shared values and social norms that build trust, group identity, and group efficacy with "safety as the priority" are essential for creating cultures of safety.

Social hierarchies also have an effect on team conflict and collaboration. Health care organizations demonstrate unique social hierarchies. Because of the dominance of the professions of medicine (which goes considerably beyond the clinical realm) and management, the communication practices, conflict, collaboration, and displays of emotions are profoundly affected. The "professionalization" of management has contributed to the complexity of the health care organization and can lead to team ineffectiveness through its diversity of education, professional socialization that competes for professional dominance and finite resources (Clement, 2001). Conflict tends to escalate in diverse and stressful environments, leading to interdisciplinary and interdepartmental communication failures and conflict, which include dissatisfaction, disagreement, or unmet expectations. This diversity, however, can also lead to a better understanding of complex systems when multiple views contribute to a more comprehensive picture of the situation. Unless conflict utilization strategies deal with the underlying structures, however, they are often unsuccessful. It is like rearranging the chairs on the Titanic. While there is plenty of activity by plenty of people, the fundamental problems are not addressed and the outcomes do not change.

Managers have a profound effect on intradepartmental team effectiveness through their behavior and relationships. Edmondson's research of organizational factors that account for variance in drug error rates across hospital units suggested that detected error rates were a function of at least two influences:

(1) actual errors made, and (2) unit members' willingness to report errors. Higher error rates and interdisciplinary collaboration were reported in units where the nurse manager scored higher in direction setting, coaching, perceived unit performance outcomes, and quality relationships. This counterintuitive relationship to errors, however, suggests that a primary influence on detected error rates is the unit members' willingness to discuss mistakes openly. This willingness may be due to leadership behavior that establishes a climate of openness and facilitates dialogue. In units with authoritarian styles and climates, there is a significant decrease in willingness to collaborate across professions and report errors (Edmondson, 1996).

The medical profession has a significant effect on team collaboration in the hospital setting. Collaboration implies an interaction that is complementary, with input and responses from each participant allowing for synergistic building to promote patient care (Baggs, 1998). While collaborative practice is talked about (mostly by nurses), research indicates that only 14% of physicians and 7% of nurses reported using collaborative interdisciplinary problem-solving approaches. The most common modes used by both providers were competition and avoidance. The staff nurses' role in clinical decision-making was more supportive than collaborative, with physicians accepting nurses' input but handling final decision-making (Forte, 1997). Many nurses do not want more responsibility than this, however. Thus, the obstacles to collaborative practice come from both the nursing and medical professions.

Teamwork Strategies: Practical Application

Briefings.   The number one teamwork goal is to create environments that promote and reward open communication and teamwork. Numerous strategies and courage are needed to change the culture of the organization from hierarchical and autonomous practice to collaborative practice through a team approach. Therefore, strategies that bring people together around the core business of patient care are practical starting points.

A briefing is a structured type of interaction used to attain clear, timely, and effective communication (Leonard, Graham, & Taggart, 2004). When briefings are structured into the day and/or processes, critical information can be shared concisely and effectively, providing just-in-time information to monitor and correct situations. Examples of briefings include: (1) "time outs" before a surgical procedure, required by the Joint Commission, to double check key risks associated with a surgical procedure such as patient identity and identification of the correct procedure; and (2) "time outs" during a hectic day on a nursing unit to identify key risks and develop a plan to intervene and support quickly and effectively.

In nursing units, briefings during shift change, patient transfer, and hand-offs in general are critical to avoid information loss in the transition.

Physician–Nurse Interaction Tool.   Nurses often feel unprepared to communicate information to physicians in a clear and concise fashion, especially in the middle of the night or when physicians have a tendency to act impatient. The Institute of Healthcare Improvement recommends a tool for the purpose of improving physician–nurse interaction: the SBAR (situation, background, assessment, and recommendation) tool. This template, outlined in Table 7.5, can be used to assist the nurse in his or her critical thinking by setting the expectations for communication of specific informational elements.

When used as the standard for communication, the SBAR model can be a very effective tool for the care team as it helps the nurse to set the expectation

Table 7.5 The SBAR Template for Nurse–Physician Communication

S	Situation	I am calling about: The patient's code status is: The problem I am calling about is: I have just assessed the patient personally: Vital signs are: I am concerned about the:
B	Background	The patient's mental status is: The skin is: The patient is not or is on oxygen.

A	Assessment	This is what I think the problem is:
		The problem seems to be: cardiac infection/
		  neurologic/respiratory.
		I am not sure what the problem is, but the patient
		  is deteriorating.
		The patient seems to be unstable and may get worse.
		  We need to do something.

R	Recommendation	I suggest or request that you:
		Are any tests needed, such as:
		If a change in treatment is ordered, then ask about their
		  next expectations for monitoring, calling, duration of
		  symptoms.

Source: Adapted with permission from copyrighted material of Kaiser Foundation Health Plan, Inc., California Regions.

of gathering information before the conversation, critically think through the information, and provide clear recommendations for care that are relevant to the patient's current condition.

Integration of this tool into nursing curriculums, orientation, professional development, and case reviews is also an effective way to decrease variability in communication and enhance patient care management.

Anticipate the Unexpected

Human fallibility and errors were pervasive and foreseeable in numerous studies of large-scale disasters; for example, the nuclear power plant explosion at Chernobyl, the 1986 Challenger space shuttle explosion shortly after take-off, and the 1979 Three Mile Island nuclear meltdown. What was not pervasive, however, were well-developed systems, processes, and skills to detect and contain errors at their early stages.

A change of thinking is required if health care organizations are to become more resilient and move beyond prevention to include cure. "To be resilient is to be mindful about errors that have already occurred and to correct them before they worsen and cause serious harm" (Weick & Sutcliffe, 2001, p. 67). Error and practice breakdown often occur when the unexpected is encountered. The skills related to noticing, coping, and correcting are very different from the skills needed for planning and anticipating. Both sets of skills are necessary.

Health care organizations often anticipate errors through the development of copious policies and procedures. Policies and procedures have their virtues, which include removing some uncertainty, promoting interdepartmental coordination, providing a pretext for learning, protecting individuals against blame, and discouraging private informal modifications. However, a wholehearted commitment to anticipation is also dangerous (Wildavsky, 1991). It presumes a level of simplicity and understanding that is impossible to achieve when dealing in complex situations. It gives people the illusion that they have things under control, and it can actually result in more complexity and opaqueness with each added policy or procedure.

This climate of anticipation in health care organizations consumes great quantities of resources and attention. Solutions to anticipated problems are created with the expectation that the group will actively retain them in their action repertoire and memory. The pre-designed solutions are then considered to be available for accessing and applied to any problem that arises.

One antidote to this obsession with planning is experiential learning. Experiential learning is being open to having one's expectations refined, challenged, or disconfirmed by the unfolding situation. Patient care involves much uncertainty. When certainty is missing (as in situations that are ambiguous), somewhat undetermined, unexpected, or markedly different than one's preconceptions, thinking and judgment are required to act (Benner et al., 1999). Resilience comes through experiential learning during and following those times of uncertainty as well as through conceptual slack, or the willingness to question what is happening rather than feign understanding.

Anticipating the unexpected is enhanced through human factor and reliability science, which is the science of evidence-based design that takes human factors (such as fatigue, distractions, interruptions, cognitive shortcomings, and emotional tendencies), and applies system design principles for failure prevention, identification, and mitigation.

Anticipation: Practical Application

Health care organizations can enhance patient-care practitioners' ability to anticipate through evidence-based design and standardization. Health care environments are laden with individual-based preferences of practice, as well as distractions and stressors that make it very difficult for practitioners to anticipate and focus (Scott, 2004). Rather than a primary focus on retrospective attentional deficits, health care organizations can focus on clear expectations through evidence-based standardization. To expect everyone to remember everything is no longer realistic. When health care designers create systems that require standardization and adherence, such as required fields in electronic medical records, and/or integrate attentional tools, such as monitor alarms that communicate directly to the bedside nurse, the system is far easier to control and reliability is enhanced.

Concerted efforts must also be made to identify and minimize distractions and stressors in the environment. For example, designing areas for medication dispensing and review that are quiet and private rather than in heavy traffic areas greatly decreases the distractions that are so often the precursors to medication errors and enhances safe medication administration.

Leaders are responsible for intentional planning and implementation of evidence-based design strategies to maximize standardization, redundancy, and critical failure mode functions as well as to monitor process compliance and results.

Defer to Expertise

HROs have mastered the ability to alter the typical patterns of deference as the tempo of operations changes and unexpected problems arise. Rather than status and rank determining who made the decisions, expertise is the determining factor. An expert is the person(s) with the best knowledge of the current situation. They have a focus and understanding of the most salient issues, are able to recognize the unexpected, and develop new knowledge of the situation. In clinical scenarios this is often the nurse at the bedside. He or she is focused on the patient and understands the subtle changes using tacit and conscious knowledge.

The patient and/or their significant others should also be considered experts and need to be integrated adequately into the systems we are striving to change (The National Patient Safety Foundation's Patient and Family Advisory Council, 2003). Patients understand their bodies in ways that health care practitioners never will, and their participation in care as well as their family members/significant others is a critical factor in keeping them safe. To build these partnerships, a fundamental shift in thinking is needed that moves health care organizations from being practitioner-centered to patient/family-centered.

In the health care industry, multiple and rapid changes are approved at the executive level often without the benefit of a clinical perspective. As a result, care delivery systems have been altered in ways that hinder or delay patient care (Benner et al., 1999). Many systems have gone through re-engineering efforts where discrete functions, tasks, and goals have been identified and designed into the system, but the broad integrative functions and knowledge work required for reliability and problem solving at the point of service were overlooked. System design approaches have focused on efficiency and recurring problems, rather than the practices, contingencies, and reliability created by the frontline problem solvers (Benner et al., 1999).

By blending a hierarchical decision structure with a specialist decision structure at the unit and organizational levels, health care organizations are able to operationalize decision-making by those with the experience and expertise. The decision-makers migrate up and down the hierarchical structure, depending on the issue, accountability, responsibility, uniqueness of the problem, and environmental characteristics (Weick & Sutcliffe, 2001).

Deferring to Expertise: Practical Application

Critical Rescue Team.   A critical rescue or rapid response team is a team created and trained to act as a self-correcting performance unit to counteract the ever-present potential for bad patient outcomes. Anyone can initiate the call to convene the on-call team for rapid convergence. The team quickly assembles to provide a second set of eyes, second opinion, a focused dialogue, and/or direct assistance to the nurse and patient. Triggers to initiate the team can be anything from staff uneasiness about a patient's condition, to a change in heart rate, systolic blood pressure, respiratory rate, oxygenation, or level of consciousness. The goal is to intervene in the patient's decline early enough to turn the situation around; this is evidenced by a decrease in cardiac arrests, ICU transfers, and patient mortality.

The team members are those with expertise in unstable patient conditions—that is, a critical care nurse, respiratory therapist, intensivist, and pharmacist—and expertise in interpersonal skills. It is critical that the team members are respectful and nonjudgmental when consulting, supporting the clinicians and others involved in the situation. This requires clear expectations and training as well as feedback from those who utilize the services.

Evidence-Based Standards Through Shared Decision-Making.   Through the creation of structures that bring situational and content experts to the table to make decisions, evidence-based standards and practices can be developed and implemented for managing and leading nurses as well as for the clinical work of nursing. Many of the profession's current practices (clinical and managerial) are based on tradition and are perpetuated without question. Structures are needed that bring the experts together in ways that enable them to voice their concerns as well as understand and own the issues that they have the expertise to change. This understanding includes the necessity of seeing the connections to the whole organization as well as the power to influence the system.

Behavioral, organizational, and reliability research has identified management practices that are consistently associated with successful implementation of change initiatives and achievement of safety in spite of high risk for error. The HRO framework is an evidence-based management structure to guide nursing leaders' work. Through planned leadership and action, organizations can accomplish the changes required in nurses' work environments to minimize variability and improve patient safety.

Evidence-based nursing standards are needed to minimize the variation of practice. Standards focused on the key activities of direct-care nursing will enhance patient outcomes and the practice of nursing. Key nursing activities for organizations to focus on for standard development are monitoring of patient status (surveillance); physiologic/disease interventions; compensation for patient's loss of functioning; provision of emotional support; patient and family education; delegation and supervision; and communication, coordination, and integration of care.

Patients and Family Members as Experts.   To change the culture of health care organizations to become patient/family centered rather than practitioner centered, several actions have been identified by the National Patient Safety Foundation (2003). These include:

1. Teaching and encouraging effective communication skills for both patients/families and health care professionals.

2. Engaging leadership in promoting and training providers in open communication about medical error (disclosure).
3. Empowering hospital patient representatives to effectively advocate and facilitate communication for patients and families during and following practice breakdown and/or medical error.
4. Establishing patient and family advisory councils to ensure a patient/family perspective is represented in all aspects of health care delivery.

This change in thinking requires strong leadership at the unit and executive levels of the organization.

Extra-Sensitive to Operations

The term "operations" is defined as the performance of the practical work within the organization that produces the "output" of patient care. HROs elevate the value of day-to-day operations above the strategic planning and administrative functions. Prestige flows to the experts at the point of service, rather than primarily to the senior leaders and planners. HROs' hierarchies or bureaucracies do not promote dysfunction. Rather, they promote high interaction and communication flow to "enhance situational awareness" through connection of the big picture and current operations (Weick & Sutcliffe, 2001). This connection requires a more holistic view for planners and practitioners alike.

Sensitivity to operations requires paying attention to the subtle symptoms and elimination of "hopeful" thinking. Hoping a problem goes away when working in a high-risk environment is not conducive to reliable patient outcomes. Nor is the human tendency to disconfirm evidence that does not fit within one's particular paradigm. Through a commitment to effective measures, timely interdisciplinary and interdepartmental dialogue, and active listening, organizational members' understanding of the complexities are deepened and enriched for early problem identification and early action.

Measures have a significant effect on the management of and behavior related to variability and reliability. Initiatives to reward employees for the best safety records, for example, often build in the incentive to withhold information about small accidents and near-misses, resulting in an actual increase in unsafe activities. Likewise, measures of safety in health care organizations imposed by third parties can miss the mark and encourage behaviors that reinforce poor performance and errors, rather than reduce them. The logic of many third-party regulations is that the presence of certain qualifying criteria or processes will be correlated to safe and effective care. However, this is often a fallacy. It is important for leaders to develop metrics to measure the most common practice breakdowns and failures; these measures should go beyond clinical process measures and include a balance of outcome metrics that are representative of the interrelatedness of the whole (i.e., productivity measures in parallel with clinical outcome measures).

Operations Sensitivity: Practical Application

Tests of Change.   Available evidence shows that most public and private organizations can be significantly improved at an acceptable cost, but that often terrible mistakes are made when this is tried, because history has not prepared the change agents for transformational challenges (Kotter, 1996). A "test of change" is defined as a small scale iterative process of the Plan-Do-Study-Act (PDSA) cycle, with each cycle leading directly into the start of the next. It is experiential organizational learning, a type of learning process in which the organizational members who generate the data are involved in the interpretation and understand the context in which the test of change exists. Therefore, it is important that the new information generated through the iterative process is shared with the individuals involved and that the collective interpretation of the new information is acted upon by the group. The follow-up action serves both to test the interpretation and to generate new information to continue the learning (Figure 7.1).

Trigger Audits.   The use of "triggers" to identify adverse events is a useful and effective method for measuring the overall level of harm from medications and other high-risk events in health care organizations. "Trigger audits" are defined as retrospective reviews of patient records using high-risk triggers to identify possible adverse events rather than depend on voluntary reporting and tracking of standard variance, practice breakdown, and error.

Figure 7.1   Linking Tests of Change

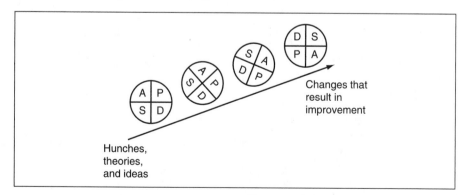

Source: From the Institute of Healthcare Improvement Web site, 2004. Reprinted with permission.

The Institute for Healthcare Improvement (IHI) in partnership with Premier, Inc. has developed a trigger tool for measuring adverse drug events (ADEs). The tool, available on the IHI Website (www.ihi.org), includes a list of known ADE triggers and instructions for measuring the number and degree of harmful medication events, and provides instructions to measure ADEs per 1,000 doses and percent of admissions with an ADE.

The concept of triggers goes beyond medication administration, however. Health care leaders and quality managers can identify triggers related to any risk process and conduct audits to determine the reliability of care in the organization. Triggers to inform nursing practice are many, as shown in Table 7.6.

Trigger audits are effective ways for health care leaders to identify contributors to events that can and do cause harm to patients, so that error can be prevented or mitigated.

Reluctance to Simplify

"Reluctance to simplify" has its roots in recognizing one's assumptions and expectations as well as in recognizing the human tendency to disconfirm evidence that does not meet one's expectations (Weick & Sutcliffe, 2001). The an-

Table 7.6 Failure Mode Triggers for Evaluating Nursing Care

1. Positive blood culture
2. Patient fall
3. Decubiti
4. Restraint use
5. Transfer to a higher level of care
6. Respiratory arrest
7. Narcan (naloxone) use
8. Oversedation/hypotension
9. Hospital-acquired pneumonia
10. Unintentional extubation

tidote to the simplification tendency is a mindful style of managing and practicing. Mindfulness preserves the capability to see the significant meaning of weak signals and to give strong responses to weak signals versus the more intuitive act of responding only to the more obvious pitfalls and dangers.

Reluctance to simplify represents an understanding of the necessity of studying variability and deficiencies not in isolation, but as embedded in its system with many links and variables, or interdependencies, which are recognized by their effects on one another and on themselves (Dörner, 1987; Reason, 1990). Understanding interdependency requires new methods of inquiry that are distinct from analysis. It requires systems thinking.

Analysis is a three-step process that first takes apart that which it seeks to understand. Then it attempts to explain the behavior of the parts taken separately. Finally, it tries to aggregate understanding of the parts into an explanation of the whole. This linear view suggests a simple locus of responsibility. When things go wrong, there is an assumption that there must be an individual, or individual agent, responsible (Senge, 1990).

A systems-thinking approach uses a different process than analysis. It puts the system in the context of the larger environment of which it is a part and studies the role it plays on the larger whole (Gharajedaghi, 1999). Peter Senge (1990) identifies several generic structures, or archetypes, that embody the key to learning so that the structures in organizations can be seen that simplify the complexity of many management issues and resistance can be leveraged and overcome. These key structures often found in many feedback processes are (1) reinforcing feedback, (2) balancing feedback, and (3) delays.

Reinforcing feedback involves processes that amplify the situation, producing more movement in the same direction, such as financial incentives for goal attainment. Balancing feedback involves processes that stabilize a situation, thus maintaining the status quo. Balancing processes are everywhere in complex systems, but are more difficult to see than reinforcing loops, especially when there are delays in the system. Balancing processes underlie all goal-oriented behavior, such as temperature regulation of the human body, or medication-error reduction. The balancing process maintains the status quo even when all participants want change. For example, when organizations create processes to decrease medication-administration errors, the actual training, monitoring, and information technology may reinforce or accelerate error reduction. On the other hand, there are balancing processes that continue the status quo, such as cultures that blame and staffing practices. Rather than pushing harder to overcome resistance to change, artful leaders discern the source of the resistance through focusing directly on the implicit norms and power relationships in which the norms are embedded (Senge, 1990). In the medication example, the leader could identify barriers to open reporting and dialogue related to errors, such as sanctions and discipline, or re-evaluate staffing based on medication administration volume.

In health care, there has been a strong movement toward simplification through standardization of the work through clinical protocols and care pathways. Reliable and standardized patient care, however, is dependent upon an understanding of the complexity of the objective and subjective system within which it exists.

Resisting the Urge to Simplify: Practical Application

Incident Reviews.   Health care leaders can understand the fundamental/root contributors to system and practice breakdown through conducting timely (within 24 hours) incident reviews that go beyond the root-cause analysis approach of problem solving to include a whole-systems thinking approach. This approach examines the more obvious objective behaviors, systems, and processes as well as the more subjective team dynamics, human interactions, underlying norms, values, and beliefs. Table 7.7 presents selected items from an "error-event interview guide" that probes the objective and subjective contributors to an error-event that potentially resulted in harm to a patient. The guide is composed of 27 questions that explore key emotional intelligence skills identified through research (Scott, 2004), using the emotional intelligence quotient Map of Cooper and Sawaf (1996) and the HRO framework as a guide. It is critical to involve the individuals who contributed to an error event in the interview process not only for their insights, but also for their feedback and learning for future error mitigation and/or management.

Through partnering with risk managers and legal counsel, health care leaders must come to consensus on processes for candid assessment and disclosure of practice breakdown so that learning can occur throughout the organization. Through the development of a consistent approach using a structured plan that digs deep and unearths the fundamental problems, strategies can be leveraged for more effective results.

CONCLUSIONS

Health care organizations are complex, encumbered with goals and information that are often ambiguous and uncertain, and with rapid changes that are communicated to and through many people during stressful times. The environment's uncertainty and complexity limit the attention and working memory of providers as well as their problem-solving abilities.

Health care organizations must become highly reliable to regain the trust of the public, patients, and patient care providers. Creating environments and structures that put patient safety first is a paradigmatic shift that will evolve through focused strategies derived from an evidence-based, reliability framework.

Table 7.7   Selected Items from Scott's Error-Event Interview Guide

The Work Itself and an Overall Description of the Event

1. Tell me about your role and responsibilities in the organization.
2. Describe the event that happened on (date) from your perspective.
3. What explanation do you have for why the error occurred?

Culture

1. How would you describe the culture you currently work in, with culture defined as the norms and expectations of those whom you work with?
2. Is this culture you are describing unique to your area only, or is it found elsewhere in the organization?
3. What significant change or changes related to attitudes and/or behaviors would you recommend to hospital leadership that would promote a culture of patient safety?

Work Pressures (at the time of incident)

1. Describe your relationship with your immediate supervisor at the time of the incident.
2. Describe your relationship with the individual(s) you were communicating with around the time the incident occurred.
3. Describe your workload/assignment the day of the incident.

Emotional Self-Awareness

1. Describe your feelings before-during-after the incident.

Emotional Expression

1. How do you feel when you are called upon to express an opinion?

Emotional Awareness of Others

1. Describe your perception of how the person you were interacting with was feeling at the time of your discussion.

Constructive Discontent

1. Describe how you usually handle difficult situations, i.e., when you disagree with someone else about something important to you.
2. How did you handle disagreement with others in the time around the incident (if applicable)?

Trust Radius

1. What about on the day of the incident? Did you feel you could ask questions, disagree, provide input, problem-solve freely (if appropriate)?

Source: Used with permission from unpublished dissertation: *Errors and Failures in Complex Health-Care Systems: Individual, Team, System and Cultural Contributors*, by K. A. Scott, 2004. Adapted with permission.

Through approaching the work of patient care from a new place—a place that acknowledges human facilities, re-examines discarded information, monitors expectations through a reliability lens, and consciously removes ineffective thinking and replaces it with evidence-based systems thinking—the very foundation of health care will be transformed.

REFERENCES

Alderfer, C. (1987). An intergroup perspective on group dynamics. In J. W. Lorsch (Ed.), *Handbook of Organizational Behavior.* Englewood Cliffs, NJ: Prentice Hall.

Argyris, C. (1985). Interventions for improving leadership effectiveness. *Journal of Management Development, 4*(5), 30–50.

Argyris, C. (1990). *Overcoming Organizational Defenses.* Boston, MA: Allyn & Bacon.

Argyris, C. (1991). Teaching smart people how to learn. *Harvard Business Review, 69*(3), 99–109.

Aroskar, M. (1985). Ethical relationships between nurses and physicians: Goals and realities—a nursing perspective (pp. 44–62). In A. Bishop & J. Scudder (Eds.), *Caring, Curing, Coping.* Tuscaloosa, AL: The University of Alabama Press.

Baggs, J. G. (1998). Nurse-physician collaboration: The challenge of collaboration. In A. L. Suchman, R. J. Botelho, & P. Hinton-Walker (Eds.), *Partnerships in Healthcare: Transforming Relational Process* (pp. 185–197). Rochester, NY: University of Rochester Press.

Becher, E., & Chassin, M. (2001). Improving quality, minimizing error: Making it happen. *Health Affairs, 20*(3), 68–81.

Benjamin, G. (2000). Addressing medical errors: The key to a safer health care system. *Physician Executive, 26*(2), 66–67.

Benner, P., Hooper-Kyriakidis, P., & Stannard, D. (1999). *Clinical Wisdom and Interventions in Critical Care.* Philadelphia, PA: W. B. Saunders.

Benner, P., Tanner, C., & Chesla, C. (1996). *Expertise in Nursing Practice: Caring, Clinical Judgment, and Ethics.* New York, NY: Springer-Verlag.

Chassin, M., & Galvin, R. (1998). The urgent need to improve health care quality: Institute of Medicine national roundtable on health care quality, consensus statement. *Journal of the American Medical Association, 280*(11), 1000–1005.

Clement, J. (2001). The leadership imperative: Managing conflict and resolving disputes creatively. *Seminars for Nurse Managers, 9*(4), 211–217.

Cohen, E., & Gooch, J. (1990). *Military Misfortunes: The Anatomy of Failure in War.* New York, NY: Vintage Books, Random House.

Coile Jr., R. C. (2001). Quality pays: A case for improving clinical care and reducing medical errors. *Healthcare Trends, 46*(3), 156–160.

Cooper, R., & Sawaf, A. (1996). *Executive EQ: Emotional Intelligence in Leadership and Organizations.* New York, NY: Berkley Publishing Group, Penguin Publishing Inc.

Coutu, D. (2003, April). Sense and reliability. *Harvard Business Review,* 84–90.

Cox, K. (2003). The effects of intrapersonal, intragroup, and intergroup conflict on team performance effectiveness and work satisfaction. *Nursing Administration Quarterly, 27*(2), 153–163.

Deming, W. (1986). *Out of the Crisis*, 2nd ed. Cambridge, MA: Massachusetts Institute of Technology.

Dixon, N. (1999). *The Organizational Learning Cycle: How We Can Learn Collectively*, 2nd ed. Cambridge, UK: Cambridge University Press.

Dörner, D. (1987). On the difficulties people have in dealing with complexity. In J. Rasmussen, K. Duncan & J. Leplat (Eds.), *New Technology and Human Errors*. London, UK: Wiley.

Dörner, D. (1996). *The Logic of Failure: Recognizing and Avoiding Error in Complex Situations*. New York, NY: Metropolitan Books.

Druskat, V., & Wolff, S. (2001, March). Building the emotional intelligence of groups. *Harvard Business Review*, 81–90.

Edmondson, A. (1996, March). Learning from mistakes is easier said than done: Group and organizational influences on the detection and correction of human error. *Journal of Applied Behavioral Science*, *32*(1), 5–28.

Forster, A., Murff, H., Peterson, J., Gandhi, T., & Bates, D. (2003). The incidence and severity of adverse events affecting patients after discharge from the hospital. *Annals of Internal Medicine*, *138*(3), 161–167.

Forte, P. (1997). The high cost of conflict. *Nursing Economic$*, *15*(3), 119–123.

Fountain, R. (1999). *The Relationship of Error-Based Experiential Learning to Organizational Change: How and Why What We Learn May or May Not Change How We Behave*. Unpublished doctoral dissertation. Cleveland, OH: Case-Western Reserve University.

Foushee, H., Lauber, J., Baetge, M., & Acomb, D. (1986). *Crew Factors in Flight Operations III: The Operational Significance of Exposure to Short-Haul Air Transport Operations*. Technical Memorandum No. 88342. Moffett Field, CA: NASA-Ames Research Center.

Gharajedaghi, J. (1999). *Systems Thinking: Managing Chaos and Complexity*. Woburn, MA: Butterworth-Heinemann.

Goleman, D. (1998). *Working with Emotional Intelligence*. New York, NY: Bantam Books.

Goleman, D. (2000, March-April). Leadership that gets results. *Harvard Business Review*, 78–90.

Grube, A. (2001). Learning from healthcare errors: Effective reporting systems. *Journal for Healthcare Quality*, *23*(1), 25–29.

Hackman, J. (1987). The design of work teams. In J.W. Lorsch (Ed.), *Handbook of Organizational Behavior* (pp. 315–342). Englewood Cliffs, NJ: Prentice Hall.

Helmreich, R. (2003, October 3). Culture, threat, and error: Lessons from aviation. Paper presented at the 2003 Seventh Annual Magnet Conference, Houston, Texas.

Institute of Healthcare Improvement. Available at http://www.ihi.org/IHI/Topics/Reliability/ReliabilityGeneral/. Retrieved March 2005.

Institute of Medicine and Kohn, L. T., Corrigan, J. M., & Donaldson, M. S. (Eds.). (1999). *To Err Is Human: Building a Safer Health System*. Washington, DC: National Academy Press.

Institute of Medicine, Committee on Quality of Health Care in America. (2004). *Keeping Patients Safe: Transforming the Work Environment of Nurses*. Washington, DC: National Academy Press.

Institute of Medicine, Committee on Quality of Health Care in America. (2001). *Crossing the Quality Chasm: A New Health System for the 21st Century*. Washington, DC: National Academy Press.

Klein, R., Bigley, G., & Roberts, K. (1995). Organizational culture in high reliability organizations: An extension. *Human Relations*, *48*(7), 771–793.

Kotter, J. (1996). *Leading Change*. Boston, MA: Harvard Business School Press.

Leape, L. (1999). The causes and prevention of errors and adverse events in health care. *Image: Journal of Nursing Scholarship, 31*(3), 281–286.

Leape, L. (1994). Error in medicine. *Journal of the American Medical Association, 272*(23), 1851–1857.

Leonard, M., Frankel, A., Simmonds, T., & Vega, K. (2004). *Achieving Safe and Reliable Healthcare: Strategies and Solutions.* Chicago, IL: Health Administration Press.

Leonard, M., Graham, S., & Taggart, B. (2004). The human factor: Effective teamwork and communication in patient strategy. In M. Leonard, A. Frankel, T. Simmonds, & K. Vega (Eds.), *Achieving Safe and Reliable Healthcare: Strategies and Solutions* (pp. 37–64). Chicago, IL: Health Administration Press.

Linking tests of change. Available at http://www.ihi.org/IHI/Topics/Improvement/Improvement Methods/How ToImprove/ramp/. Retrieved March 2005.

Lovallo, D., & Dahneman, D. (2003, July). Delusions of success: How optimism undermines executives' decisions. *Harvard Business Review,* 56–63.

Malloch, K., & Porter-O'Grady, T. (2005). *The Quantum Leader: Applications for the New World of Work.* Sudbury, MA: Jones and Bartlett.

Mayer, B. (2000). *The Dynamics of Conflict Resolution: A Practitioner's Guide.* San Francisco, CA: Jossey-Bass.

Merriam-Webster's Collegiate Dictionary, 10th ed. (2002). Springfield, MA: Merriam-Webster, Inc.

Merry, M., & Brown, J. (2002). From a culture of safety to a culture of excellence: Quality science, human factors, and the future of healthcare quality. *Journal of Innovative Management, 7*(2), 29–46.

Perrow, C. (1984). *Normal Accidents: Living with High Risk Technologies.* New York, NY: Basic Books.

Pronovost, P., Angus, D., Dorman, T., Robinson, K., Dremsizov, T., & Young, T. (2002). Physician staffing patterns and clinical outcomes in critically ill patients: A systematic review. *Journal of the American Medical Association, 288*(17), 2151–2162.

Reason, J. (2000, March). Human error: Models and management. *British Medical Journal, 320*(7237), 768–770.

Reason, J. (1990). *Human Error.* New York, NY: Cambridge University Press.

Rovner, J. (2000). Washington wakes up to medical mistakes. *Business & Health, 18*(11), 19.

Sagan, S. (1993). *The Limits of Safety: Organizations, Accidents, and Nuclear Weapons.* Princeton, NJ: Princeton University.

Scott, K. (2004). Errors and failures in complex health-care systems: Individual, team, system and cultural contributors. Unpublished dissertation. Cincinnati, OH: The Union Institute & University.

Senge, P. (1990). *The Fifth Discipline: The Art and Practice of the Learning Organization.* New York, NY: Doubleday.

Sexton, J., Thomas, E., & Helmreich, R. (2000, March). Error, stress, and teamwork in medicine and aviation: Cross sectional surveys. *British Medical Journal, 320*(7237), 745–749.

Shi, L., & Singh, D. (2001). *Delivering Health Care in America: A Systems Approach.* Gaithersburg, MD: Aspen Publishers.

Smith, M., & Forster, H. (2000). Morally managing medical mistakes. *Cambridge Quarterly of Healthcare Ethics, 9*(1), 38–53.

The National Patient Safety Foundation's Patient and Family Advisory Council. (2003). National agenda for action: Patients and families in patient safety: Nothing about me, without me. North Adams, MA: The National Patient Safety Foundation.

Weick, K. (1990). The vulnerable system: An analysis of the Tenerife air disaster. *Journal of Management, 16*(3), 571–593.

Weick, K., & Sutcliffe, K. (2001). *Managing the Unexpected: Assuring High Performance in an Age of Complexity.* San Francisco, CA: Jossey-Bass.

Wildavsky, A. (1991). *Searching for Safety.* New Brunswick, NJ: Transaction Publishers.

CHAPTER 8

Partnership Economics: Creating Value Through Evidence-Based Workload Management

Tim Porter-O'Grady and Kathy Malloch

There is much concern these days regarding the availability and productivity of nursing resources. With nurses in short supply, interest is accelerating the effort to address the economics and resource implications of nursing in the health care system (Horak, Welton, & Shortell, 2004). Much has been written about the economic issues and impact of this nursing shortage as it relates to the crisis for efficient, effective, and profitable health care organizations (Buerhaus, 1991).

While the supply and demand issues of nursing are certainly important, it is interesting to note that they become of general interest only when nurses are in short supply. When the supply issues are addressed and the nursing shortage no longer appears critical, nursing moves off the priority agenda of most health care leadership, descending down the ladder of operational or economic importance (Beurhaus, 1995). Because of this diminishing focus on nursing resources, many hospitals forget their core business, which sometimes has even crippled their business and strategic viability (Hope, 2004).

Nursing has a colorful history of oppressed group dynamics (Ashley, 1976). Clearly, the fact that nursing historically has been a predominantly female profession in a subservient role has had a tremendous influence on the role, power, and position of nursing within the health care system. Two major barriers have affected the development of nursing: the first—and most obvious—is the feminine predominance on the development of the profession. Secondly, the dominating political and economic development of medicine as a social script, supported and encouraged by the servile role of nurses, has predominated in the development of the health care system (Butterworth, 1979). As a result, most nurses have been managed, controlled, and limited by the dominating lay management and medical system (Starr, 1984).

Simultaneously, as a masculine medically dominated health care system emerged, the nursing resource silently, yet steadily, became central to the clinical

183

and service efficacy of the system. Because of the need to have competently educated practitioners available to patients 24 hours a day, a growing commitment to the education, development, and role impact of nursing created an insidious and central role for the nurse in the delivery of clinical services. Parallel to this important role, an equally insidious infrastructure has developed that is represented by tight control, significant and detailed regulation, and precisely defined parameters for clinical decision-making, dependence on authority, and independence (Kalisch & Kalisch, 2003). While nurses have become increasingly well educated and advances in clinical practice have unfolded consistent with the increase in the complexity of clinical service, the challenges of control and influence remain. Among such circumstances as inadequate resource planning, limited inclusion of nurses in strategic and policy decisions, financial and economic decisions made without nursing consultation, and external improvements in choice and opportunity for women, the shortage of nurses has regularly, and with increasing intensity, become common in the health care system (Buerhaus & Needleman, 2000). Again, it is at these times that the importance and central value of nursing becomes most visible to leaders in the health care and political system. Significant efforts at increasing the numbers and recruiting women (and some men) into the profession to address care needs operate at a frenzied level. However, significantly little is done to alter the power position, practice parameters, and long-term financial condition of nurses and nursing (including nursing educators), all of which have been indicated by nurses as central to their need for satisfaction and continuing interest in the profession (Traynor, 1999).

Together these factors challenge the economic, social, and political positions and conditions of nursing. Furthermore, they inform both general and specific responses to the issues of nursing finance, productivity, value, and sustainability (Moody, 2004). In fact, issues of productivity often discussed at the management and leadership level in organizations relate more to functional proficiency and basic competence determinations than they do to issues of positioning, politics, and practice (Whittmann-Price, 2004). Additionally, much of the language at the administrative level is frequently process and functionally oriented as it relates to issues of adequate numbers of nurses and appropriate levels of productivity (Eastaugh, 1998). The resulting costs in nurse dissatisfaction and job turnover are the clearest and most obvious indications of significant problems with these current functional and institutional approaches to addressing nursing resource issues (Waldman, Kelly, Arora, & Smith, 2004).

Different perceptions of the value of the nursing resource clearly must emerge in these challenging times for both nursing and health care. Furthermore, functional and institutional articulations about the value and productivity should be reflected by increased economic and financial benefits for nurses. No longer can nursing be seen simply as a functional part of the cost of doing business within a hospital or health care system context. Nursing is not merely a support or budgeted functional resource that can be managed and accounted for in the same manner as materials management. While quantification of clinical care is essential to managing financial and productivity concerns, a more evidence-based approach to determine this value and the subsequent financial representation of nurses' value must be a critical shift in focus. All too often, the reconfiguration of the financial equation in hospitals and health systems creates pressures to eliminate nursing work, which, in the end, does not result in improving economic value or improve the financial circumstances of the entire organization. Because nursing is both critical and central to the functional work of the organization, eliminating its value through sometimes arbitrary and poorly delineated decision strategies threatens the viability of the organization and ultimately affects its sustainability.

Most hospitals and health care systems today are struggling with the issue of a nursing shortage that was created by decisions on the nursing resource that were made nearly a decade ago. The hospital restructuring movement of the early 1990s created reductions in the educated nursing work force, ultimately threatening the clinical viability of the organization at the same time that clinical interventions became more complex and intense. Certainly, it is now obvious that these so-called productivity decisions of the early to mid-1990s are extracting an enormous price on the nursing resources in health care systems (Barry-Walker, 2000; Weinberg & Suzanne, 2004).

The historic lack of connection between the economic viability of the organization as it affects the satisfaction and performance of its nursing resource is an untenable factor in the future consideration of the viability of health care organizations. Administrators and other leaders in the health care system can no longer make strategic and economic decisions without recognizing how those decisions impact its primary resource: nursing. Even in an evidence-based format, managerial decisions must reflect a balancing of the value equation, that tension between service, resources, and outcomes (Malloch & Porter-O'Grady, 1999). This three-legged stool upon which clinical and performance viabilities are based becomes unbalanced when any one of the value factors is emphasized in a way that sacrifices its relationship to the other factors. Untenable and uncontrolled emphasis on providing service without consideration to issues of resource utilization creates an imbalance that ultimately affects service sustainability. Equally, a focus on producing high levels of quality without the human or financial resources to obtain and sustain that quality also creates an imbalance. Uncontrolled and overriding focus on managing cost ultimately limits and threatens the ability to provide adequate service or ensure the high quality of that service. Again, the imbalance is obvious. The economic and financial sustainability of the organization is in finding a continuous and dynamic balance between these three elements of the value equation, and keeping them in accord. Necessarily, productivity measurement must transcend to a multifaceted model that reflects the complexity of the work of nursing. This is much different than the simple and limited cost-benefit evaluation that compares work hours to budgeted units of service.

Leadership must recognize the centrality of the nursing function in order to sustain a balance in the value equation for their hospital or corporation. The nursing resource is not only the organization's largest human cost, but it is also central to the successful clinical operation of the health system. The nurse is located at the intersection of the provision of all health care services. In fact, it is the nurse's role to coordinate, integrate, and facilitate all of the clinical functions related to the delivery of patient care. Empirical evidence for "intersection management," that is, interdisciplinary coordination, is needed.

This role of intersection management clearly places the nurse in a critical position with regard to the financial and service viability of the organization. In addition, elements of high levels of quality in the delivery of clinical service are also influenced and often coordinated by nursing professionals. Nurses are the physician's "eyes and ears" to evaluate the patient's condition, response, and progress in a timely fashion. Therefore, in a high-level interface, the nurse has a direct and powerful impact on the clinical and service viability of the organization. By direct relationship, the nurse controls the financial variables that ultimately affect the economic viability of the organization (Finkler & Graf, 2001).

Organizations that recognize and build management, operational, and financial support systems for professional nursing functions in the organization actively contribute to both their service and financial variability. Administrators often argue that nursing should not be valued in a broader framework like other clinical disciplines. They forget that all other clinical disciplines value nursing by virtue of the nurses' coordination and integrative roles as they relate to their clinical actions and relationships with one another and with the patients. No specific role has greater importance than any other in health care delivery. It is vital to recognize nursing's central role, as nurses integrate all of the work of other disciplines with regard to the patients' progress along their healing continuum. This realization is the key to the clinical success of the entire health organization (While, Forbes, Ullman, Lewis, Mathes, & Grifiths, 2004).

On the other hand, it is crucial for nursing professionals to recognize that there must be a clear delineation of specific measures of value. In an evidence-based world, it is important for the nursing profession to enumerate and articulate its value in sufficiently objective terms so that real value can be identified and measured. Historically, the problem with nursing care delivery has been the difficulty to define and scientifically evaluate evidence of clinical practice at the level of performance, in a way that yields specifically delineated outcomes (Duffy, 2004). Not clearly tying practice elements and activities to specifically defined outcomes makes it exceptionally difficult to identify any unique and specified value for nursing practice. While admittedly it is extremely difficult to do because of the coordinative and integrative relationships and activities of nursing practice, it is no longer acceptable to omit that step. Nurses cannot claim value on one hand and provide little definitive evidence of that value on the other.

Reframing nursing within the context of the value equation calls the profession to critically delineate both its clinical foundations and supporting financial demands. Viable clinical practice requires that a clear foundation for that practice be delineated and accepted. Within an evidence-based context, a collective effort to establish clinical best practices calls for the consideration of several factors:

- Clearly delineated service-based protocols and practices that reflect broader best practice standards
- A professionally designed, service-specific best practice framework that incorporates generic standards into specific performance standards
- A specifically defined tie between clinical tasks, best practices, and the payment formats within which they are financed
- A real-time process that articulates clinical performance and costs of that performance within payment parameters for those clinical processes
- An infrastructure within which nursing practice is evaluated according to the context of both clinical quality and financial enumerators
- The societal mandate for nursing services based on reliable nursing knowledge
- Variance documentation as a vehicle to improve the management of resources

What is implied in building a formal process is a commitment to both the health care management system and the nursing clinical system, so that the relationship between clinical practice, performance outcomes, and the payment structure is clearly delineated (Wannisky, Centers for Medicare & Medicaid Services [U.S.], & United States, 2003). All of these factors are critical for creating a sustainable and viable relationship between the value of nursing practice, the quality of clinical outcomes, and the cost and payment factors associated with obtaining them.

In addition to creating this value foundation, it is important that the profession itself be aware of the need for a deeper understanding of the value elements of clinical practice. Too many nurses are unaware of the need to balance clinical performance against resource availability and quality outcomes. Because of the history of nursing and its predominant focus on clinical process rather than specific identification with clinical outcome, nurses have become addicted to process (Hughes & American Nurses Association, 1958). In fact, for many nurses the process has become ritual, routine, and intellectually mindless. Further, experience itself has become a mantra, even though in most cases experience tends to be a limitation. The more experience one has, the more one is inculcated in the values that experience provides (Smith, 2002). Competent practice is changing practice. As technology enhancements and innovations continually challenge the foundations of clinical practice, it is the very fluidity, flexibility, and mobility of clinical practice that ensures its continuing viability and efficacy. In this set of circumstances, nurses who continually value specific performance experience may actually limit their availability and exposure to the considerable demands for flexibility and changing practice in increasingly shorter periods of time. This blind dependence and valuing of experience over innovation and education must be overcome if meaningful value is to (1) be found, and (2) be defined (Corey, 2001).

This provides a great opportunity for building a framework for economically and financially viable evidence-based practice. The direct connection between evidence and payment must be established in order to establish a clear, direct path between nursing activity, productivity, and value. Ultimately, there must be a direct relationship between what services are paid for in health care and the percentage of that payment that relates specifically to nursing-driven activities. What is difficult in this equation is determining the value of those activities that are predominantly coordinating and integrating processes. Since this coordination and integration comprise the majority of professional nursing activity (in terms of value), it is significantly important to provide a financial relationship for it (Rubin, Plovnick, & Fry, 1975).

On the other hand, it may not be so important that individual costing and value determination provide for the specific coordinative and integrative activities of the nursing professional. In fact, what might be wiser is to determine and integrate the percentage of role and functional contribution to the integrated plan of clinical activities for each patient. Through this process, it is easier to determine the aggregated costs of service and, ultimately, break out the individual costs contributed by each discipline. In any given clinical circumstance, this percentage of contribution will be different. However, when the data are collected and analyzed, the normative distribution of time and service will emerge, thus enabling the percentage of cost allocation associated with that distribution to be normalized.

While it is important for nursing to clearly delineate its own specific functions and activities, that importance is not gained unilaterally. The value of enumerating specific professional clinical function only finds form when it is collected and integrated with the clinical activities of other associated disciplines within the context of diagnosis-related groups (DRGs). However, integration of the data first requires a clear determination of the component contribution. It is here where nursing's work is most important. In fact, it is at the level of component contribution that each discipline has specific work. Each discipline must meet five specific performance expectations before clinical integration can result in financial valuing.

1. A specific determination of professionally delineated task and performance expectations that define the unique contributions of the discipline
2. A clear enumeration of the gross cost factors associated with the human resource and functional elements of the work of the discipline
3. A clear indication of the discipline's specific and unique contribution to the clinical outcome expectations within specified patient populations
4. An ability to clearly articulate, in language that is understood and agreed upon by other disciplines, the specific performance contributions of each discipline
5. A willingness and ability to dialogue and intersect with other disciplines to build an aggregated clinical framework for specific protocols and clinical processes that best represent the contribution of each discipline to the needs of specific patient populations

Nursing will have an especially difficult time in meeting the obligations of discipline-specific definitions. The challenge for nursing is its historic commitment to the process and its lack of a clearly defined relationship to clinical outcomes. The more valuable activity for nursing in undertaking this process will be to value the time commitments related to coordinating, integrating, and facilitating the clinical work of all the disciplines, and then placing specific value on that time and effort. Important to this process on the journey to evidence-based format is attention to the following factors:

- Establishing a clear value for the nonfunctional clinical activities related to nursing performance
- Enumerating the type and character of coordinative and integrative activities fundamental to the role of the nurse
- Locating and articulating the value of nursing performance in the identified nonfunctional processes with the intersection management activities associated with nursing
- Specifically identifying those particular clinical practice standards and professional performance characteristics against which value can be established, so the outcomes indicated by them can be more clearly defined
- Distinguishing between the generic standards of practice addressing activities of the profession as a whole from those specific clinical standards that are service-, procedure-, or patient-specific
- Creating a method (formula) for determining costs and value related specifically to the clinical and coordinative activities undertaken at the point of service that reflects the standard of practice identified there

Each of these initiatives is essential for nursing (and every discipline) and is one part of identifying its technical, relational, and coordinative functions in the course of delivering patient care. Included in this process should be those team-based activities and expectations that also incorporate issues of time and relationship influencing patient outcomes and ultimately impact the financial value. Attaching financial value to the various roles and functions is the last stage of the preliminary activities of ascertaining units of value. When the discipline-specific contributions can be identified and the specific values more clearly enumerated, the aggregation and analysis of that information can provide a clear service value with a particular patient population or DRG.

To clearly delineate value, it is crucial to utilize prevailing methodology that uses payment factors as a part of value determination. Perhaps the most obvious unit of value is the DRG, since that is the predominant value unit that is used for payment in health care organizations. Evidence-based practice processes driving the formulation of protocols, standards, or best practices should be designed in a way that fits the DRG format for payment. Simply because this format is already well defined, the DRG alignment approach to clinical valuing would be useful. However, there is nothing in evidence-based practice that would require it to be the sole viable approach. Whatever approach is identified and used, it must be consistent, reducible to financial value, integrate and link the contributions of the health care disciplines, and useful as an evaluative and comparative mechanism. In addition, it should provide an opportunity to evaluate the criteria, performance, and impact of medical practice.

CREATING AN ENVIRONMENT FOR PRACTICE

In addition to establishing simple and direct values for nursing, it is equally important to recognize the value in creating a relevant environment and climate for the practice of nursing. Evidence-based practice does not unfold in isolation of the context for practice. As health care shifts in radical ways, the environment and contextual framework for practice are also shifting. Creating a healing environment for the patient in a fast-paced, short-term, highly technical frame of reference also calls for the creation of a work environment that makes it possible for nurses and other professionals to successfully render care in a different model for patient service (Institute of Medicine [U.S.] Committee on Quality of Health Care in America, & NetLibrary Inc., 2001).

This goodness-of-fit issue between the built (or physical) environment and practice is as critical to the success of practice as clarity around the elements and protocol are for care delivery. Gone are the days when environmental design included utilities and services at one end of a very long hallway, with patients needing care at the opposite end of this same hall. Also gone are the cold, sterile, and colorless environments that did not lend support to their impact on the healing process (Ulrich, Quan, Zimring, Joseph, & Choudhary, 2004).

Environments are now a critical element of the care dynamic itself, not only for patients but also for providers. Creating a management and leadership environment of engagement, openness, and valuing of the clinical provider is one aspect of the creation of an appropriate supporting structure. Other elements related to the creation of a positive work environment and increased productivity relate to the building, structural format, color, inclusion of nature, and a peaceful aesthetics. All of these factors help create a viable milieu within which to work (Ulrich et al., 2004).

The conditions of stress embedded in clinical work during a highly transforming time and equally fast-paced clinical environment have a tremendous impact on retention and turnover in clinical practice (Eberhardt, Szigeti, & University of North Dakota, 1990). Clearly, a cost-benefit analysis and review of the relationship between personal satisfaction in the exercise of clinical work and the structural environment within which it unfolds is an important corollary to supporting evidence with regards to the influence of environment. However, simply factoring the fatigue and support issues associated with environment and the practitioner is not sufficient to address the financial and economic concerns (King & Hinds, 2003). The Pebble Model/BEMC Model issues include the desirability of the environment by the patient, the market value of a healing environment to the community, and the fiscal impact of reducing length of stay, care intensity, and patient need. The Models regard creating a physical environment that facilitates healing as important as other influences on cost (Berry, Parker, Coile, Hamilton, O'Neill, & Sadler, 2004).

Furthermore, when measuring productivity and resource use, it is important that the contextual circumstances be included in the value determination. Historical work studies and other resource measurements in nursing and clinical practice have provided ample evidence about the impact of environment, structure, and support systems as it relates to the generation of clinical costs and the distribution of a clinician's time (Rice, 2000). Finding a balance between these variables, determining the financial specifics and considerations related to their impact, and incorporating them into the variable cost determination is an important methodology for ensuring the full consideration of resource use and all associated costs.

A further concern with regard to economic and financial value is the further refinements of data that lead to an increased understanding of the relationship between environment and provider risk, clinical error, and personal health and safet (Child, Institute of Medicine [U.S.], Board on Health Care Services, Committee on the Work Environment for Nurses and Patient Safety, & NetLibrary Inc., 2004). Certainly, there is a host of considerations related to the work environment and its impact on risk and safety from both the providers' and patients' perspective. These also exert a powerful impact on the cost of providing service as well as the ability to create an environment that establishes a marketable relationship between the organization and those whom it serves. Evidence exists for the close relationship between environmental issues of safety and clinical error. Knowing this, fiscal and service leaders should be able to make a clear distinction of the costs associated with these environmental and structural factors. Also, these factors should be incorporated into any of the data related to productivity and work value determinations.

At a minimum, the considerations of environment are critical to establish evidence for its influence on clinical practice as well as economics and health service costs. In building a contextual evidence-based framework for these environmental influences, the following should be considered:

- Identification of the specific healing, comfort, and patient satisfaction considerations related to the physical environment and structural context for care
- Delineation of the structural and organizational (delivery system) considerations impacting clinical practice and specific elements of work flow
- Enumeration of the impact of physical plant, environment, and structures on provider attitude, satisfaction, and turnover
- Determination of the impact of environment and structure on issues of clinical error, patient safety, and circumstances of care
- Incorporation of structural and environmental considerations in productivity measures and formulas associated with appropriate resource use and service time values

Development of an evidence-based framework to determine productivity, patient-staff ratios, clinical assignments, and provider categories is now fundamental to accurately determine value and its impact on quality and cost. (Harrington & Estes, 2004) Indeed, the accuracy of the financial data on the clinical relationship between patient and provider is now an essential construct of an appropriate, meaningful, and sustainable delivery of clinical services. Failing to include the environmental and structural considerations in the determination of productivity and clinical care not only contributes to a lack of cost control, but also further facilitates the inappropriate and possibly expensive use of unevaluated human resources.

BUILDING AN EVIDENCE-BASED FRAMEWORK

Many workload management systems are attempting to address the management and control of nursing resources. The attempt to objectively validate the distribution of staff based on the needs of care is clearly a critical measurement when defining the appropriate use of the clinical resource. However, simply looking at nursing actions and activities without reflecting on the wider number of variables does not accurately or adequately establish the evidence of their value, nor can it build a frame of reference upon which value determination can be sustained. In fact, most workload management systems for nursing have not accurately and adequately incorporated the financial and economic valuing of the contribution of the nurse from the perspective of process, structure, or outcome. Many workload management systems measure only process (time and motion) (American Nurses Association, 2000). It is clear that for effective resource management, workload systems must become evidence-based and reflect a prevailing and sustaining reality. At a minimum the following should be accomplished:

- Clearly delineate the foundations, standards, and protocols for clinical practice that relate to specific populations, DRGs, or other generally acceptable methods of patient service measurement and payment
- Link and integrate within an interdisciplinary set of standards or protocols that provide a comprehensive delineation of clinical service to the patient
- Incorporate issues of levels of expectation for clinical competence, differentiation between levels of provider, and clearly delineated performance expectations for specific patient populations or DRGs
- Obtain a more clear and strident incorporation of the structural and environmental cost factors associated with delivery of care
- Include the organizational and operational variables affecting the structure and process of care, especially those factors of the administrative infrastructure that affect the cost of delineating service
- Connect the financial, accounting, and budgeting processes of the organization to workload management and resource allocation within the context of specific clinical protocols or DRGs
- Develop, refine, and maintain a clinical resource information infrastructure for real-time data related to acuity, patient demand, resource allocation, clinical standard or protocol, structural and environmental considerations, and a continuous and effective reporting mechanism
- Be able to adjust staffing and resource allocation related to specific clinical standards, protocols, or DRG delineations in real-time as the patient's condition requires

For an effective evidence-based workload management framework to unfold, these issues must be specifically and clearly addressed. Furthermore, an integrated regional and national approach must begin to emerge in relationship to the specific appropriate measures, protocols, and standards that are applied as well as the structural and environmental considerations that are included in a workload/resource management model.

From an evidence-based practice perspective, what may be helpful when more clearly articulating nursing's value within an economic framework is the joining of interdisciplinary activities under the rubric of an integrated clinical standard of practice. Using an objective payment-related structure (such as the DRG) can provide a contextual framework within which all of the clinical disciplines can identify their contribution to the frame of reference for specific patient care protocols or processes. It is this linkage and integration among the disciplines that will create the composite framework for value determination. The evidence of impact on patient outcome, the viability of clinical process, and the cost framework that supports clinical practice can be more clearly enumerated when the disciplines speak the same language and use a common framework. However, until that time, focusing on effective nursing workload management and creating an integrated structure for valuing that work will be critical first steps toward valuing nursing practice, establishing its relationship to financial and payment concerns, and providing a baseline with which nursing resource value can be connected across the interdisciplinary health care network.

A MODEL FOR THE FUTURE

Given the complexity and inadequacies of the current measurement systems for the work of nursing caregivers, health care leaders are duly challenged to create more appropriate systems. The purpose of creating a new clinical productivity model is not to more accurately represent the work of nursing as we now know it; it is about creating a new mindset that moves leaders from expecting adequate numbers of nurses to one that focuses on achieving adequate patient care outcomes within the existing health care structure and resources. Six strategies are essential steps in the creation of a more contemporary model: (1) reframing the measurement of health care services; (2) describing the work of nursing; (3) quantifying the work of nursing in an economic model that is linked to patient outcomes; (4) embedding the new measures within existing systems; (5) evaluating performance in an aggregated model; and (6) managing the variance or system feedback to ensure system sustainability.

Reframe the Measurement of Health Care Services

New models that embrace and reflect the reality of nursing patient care services, focusing on the holistic and dynamic human condition with associated scientific, societal, and economic factors, will improve the ability of leaders to manage resources from an evidence-based perspective. In this model, the first consideration is to reconcile the separation of nursing science and nurse caring. Nursing science, which is easily represented within the economic and clinical aspects of health care, and the socially valued and essential caring dimension of nursing that is not as easily quantified must be inexorably linked and integrated into the economic system.

The first and most difficult step for health care leaders is to not only admit that the current system is not working, but also have the courage to do something about it. Patient care services continue to evolve in a technologically savvy and humanistic environment, while the measurement of these services remains embedded in basic linear principles of cause and effect based on the industrial manufacturing model. The work of nursing is ill-suited for the assembly line "widget" model for several specific reasons. These include the nonlinear work of nursing; the frequent overlapping of tasks or multitasking; interruptions from providers, families, and other patients in need of care; and the unpredictable patient priorities for pain, elimination, and nutrition. These realities of patient care require a model that embraces all of these challenges. A new model that views and measures the work of patient care from an aggregated whole rather than from disconnected tasks better represents the work of nursing in a much simpler way.

This new model also must integrate the achievement of clinical outcomes resulting from the services provided, the number of hours of care for the service, and the level of provider required to achieve these outcomes. Further, the impact of this integration is reflected in the patient care value equation in which resources, outcomes, and value are examined and evaluated, forming the philosophical foundation for a new, aggregated productivity model.

Leaders will necessarily need to modify expectations as they shift their focus from the number of hours or the quantity of work to an aggregation of resources used, resulting outcomes, and perceived value obtained. The clinical productivity model is necessarily different for nonclinical areas that do not experience the interruptions, family needs, and unpredictable patient needs for elimination, food, and comfort. Issues of multitasking are common to all employees. A new model must also include expectations for real-time data using computerized systems to guide processes of care and provide information to support process modifications in a timely manner to ensure optimal patient safety. Common definitions specific to workload management are listed in Table 8.1.

The Work of Nursing

The second consideration of the model is the work of nursing, which is described by many nurses as "providing quality nursing care," a general and

Table 8.1   Common Definitions of Nursing Workload Management

Term	Definition
Labor productivity	A measure of output divided by input; the number of units of production per hour of workload (Meyers & Stewart, 2002).
Nursing work	Includes attention to the full range of human experiences and responses to health and illness without restriction to a problem-focused orientation; integration of objective data with knowledge gained from an understanding of the patient or group's subjective experience; application of scientific knowledge to the processes of diagnosis and treatment; and provision of a caring relationship that facilitates health and healing (ANA, 2003).
Nursing productivity (traditional definition)	Ratio of output (patient care hours per patient day) to input (paid salary and benefit dollars) (O'Brien-Pallas et al., 2004).
Patient care workload	Number of patients assigned to one nurse in a specific time frame (i.e., 6 patients assigned to one nurse for this shift).
Staffing variance	Number of hours required for care is different from those available hours of staff.
Work	Effort or exertion directed to produce or accomplish something (Merriam-Webster's Collegiate Dictionary, 2002).
Workload	The amount of work that a machine, employee, or group of employees can be or is expected to perform (Merriam-Webster's College Dictionary).
Value	Relative worth or importance (Merriam-Webster's College Dictionary).

qualitative description of the service that has no quantification. Others who do not understand the work of nursing wonder if nursing is necessary with this vague and subjective description. Recent publications (Aiken, Clark, Sloane, Sochalski, & Silber et al., 2002; Needleman, Buerhaus, Mattke et al., 2002) have identified that better outcomes resulted because of nursing, and poor outcomes and patient deaths resulted from the lack of nurses. What is also lacking is the linkage between identified and specific interventions of the nurse and the health of people. The work of nursing requires objective descriptions in order to embed it in current health care measurement structures, and to link these services provided with value-based outcomes that indeed impact the quality of health. The description also requires recognition and integration of a societal mandate for nursing, the professional scope of practice, and the economic realities of the marketplace. A qualitative, descriptive overview of the work of nursing must include more than tasks that are easily observed and quantified, such as procedures and administration of medications.

Examination of nursing from the opposite side of the outcome, namely, from the time before nursing occurred or the absence of nursing as it is now known, is both illustrative and enlightening to assist in the description of nursing. When nursing is absent, it is not merely the medications that are not passed and the dressings that are not changed; much more occurs. What is lost is subtle at first, and then overwhelmingly thunderous. Patients are not monitored regularly for condition changes; failures to rescue are common and emergency codes occur; condition changes are not communicated to physicians; care is not coordinated; patient knowledge is not improved; and preventable measures such as pressure ulcers, urinary tract infections, pneumonia, and length of stay all increase.

In general, the core dimensions of the work of nursing are both physical and cognitive (Squires, 2004). These dimensions include:

- Skill performance/task management that represents the technical work of nursing. Examples include patient assessment; medication administration; intravenous access and line management; pain management; safety or restraint management; and interpreting vital signs. Note: The focus and information needed for productivity management systems are necessarily the specific interventions of the nurse rather than a description of the patient's condition. For example, identifying a "combative patient" as work to be done does not provide objective and measurable information for a clinical productivity system. However, identifying the "application of restraints and assessment every 15 minutes" provides the required information for a valid productivity system.
- Monitoring progress and oversight of patient conditions. This includes acting as the eyes and ears of physicians to prevent or manage crises.
- Evidence from the intersection management or interdisciplinary coordination of work of nursing. This includes creating and modifying plans of care in a timely manner based on patient conditions, prioritizing through analysis and synthesis of information, and coordination of the work of all disciplines caring for the patient. The work of nursing is distinct,

but necessarily embedded in an interconnected multidisciplinary model. Advocating for the patient is an integral component of interdisciplinary coordination.

- Information management. This includes knowing not only what to communicate, but to whom and when to communicate. This incorporates patient and family education as well as information management among members of the caregiver team.

- Leadership behaviors specific to the delegation and supervision of work processes. Skilled performance management of other staff; precepting new nurses.

- Relationship management. Monitoring and modifying behaviors and personalities of team members. Nurses are deeply entrenched in daily processes of relationship management with all patient care team members (physicians, nurses, managers, allied health personnel, and unlicensed assistive personnel). Experience and collective wisdom emerge from team members who work together.

Eliminate Non-Valued-Added Work

In addition to describing the work of nursing, it is also important to identify the current work of nursing that does not improve patient outcomes or provide value to the equation of care. Necessarily, the work of nursing must be integrated into the value equation in which resources and outcomes are essential elements. Providing a service merely because one is competent to perform a procedure is unacceptable when there is no measurable value to the health status of the patient. The work of nursing is about providing appropriate goal-oriented services rather than providing as many services as possible, irrespective of the cost and outcomes. Wise choices rather than rich choices for care that include fiscal implications, appropriateness of nursing care specific to outcomes, and goodness-of-fit, service quality, and patient impact are needed. The elimination of non-value-added work may be as difficult and challenging as it is to describe the work of nursing.

In Hill-Rom's study of acute care organizations, approximately 85% of the time spent by nurses was on direct and indirect activities that did not move the patient along the care path (Lanser, 2001). Murphy (2003) reported that wasteful work consumed 35% of hospital employees' time with the excessive documentation requirements, inefficient shift-to-shift or departmental reports, and searching for colleagues, supplies, and equipment. These significant percentages of non-value-added work are cause for both concern and further study. The challenge to identify the valued work is coupled with the reality that evidence is lacking to support some interventions that may indeed positively impact patient outcomes.

To be sure, nurses find it quite difficult to give up any current nursing work because all work is believed to be valuable and appropriate. The phenomenon of not being able to give up work that is believed valued in not unique to nursing. In a *Harvard Business Review* article, Johnson (2002) noted that time is the scarcest commodity—no one ever has enough—and the quality of work suffers as a result of the lack of time.

Another explanation offered by Johnson is thought provoking. The following hypothetical situation was posed to hundreds of managers, with most of them believing they already lacked the time to do their jobs properly.

A supervisor asks an employee if he or she is interested in taking on a special project. The project is of strategic importance and would provide major growth opportunities. The offer had one catch, however; the assignment is part-time and requires one day a week, which would require the individual to do the current job in four days rather than five days. Ninety-nine percent of the managers took on the assignment. These managers admitted that if the motivation was powerful enough, they could eliminate or do in much less time eight to ten hours of activities each week without negative consequences.

Would the same thing occur if nurses were given the opportunity to participate in creating a new clinical service? Could nurses in that scenario evaluate the value of their work more critically? Would giving up work actually yield untold benefits for nursing?

To begin the challenging process of eliminating non-value-added work, nurses must examine the specific nursing work that has been identified on the basis of core dimensions, professional standards, and nurse practice acts. Asking the question, "do we need this work at all," nurses should create multiple lists of tasks that should be included and things not to do anymore. Systematically and rigorously identifying and eliminating those activities that are extraneous to achieving goals further contribute to organizational effectiveness. On the other hand, eliminating interventions or work that has uncertain value without careful examination is inappropriate and can negatively impact outcomes. Structured and rigorous methods are necessary to ensure the continuing improvement in credible identification of nurse work that is based on principles of evidence-based practice. This incorporates the best research, clinical expertise, and the values of the individual members of the profession.

Non-value-added work includes both direct and indirect nurse work as well as work resulting from system inefficiencies. Examples of tasks that do not provide value to patient outcomes include:

- Patient education to those patients who are historically noncompliant. It is unrealistic to expect that an 80-year-old diabetic patient will become enlightened and change behaviors. Extensive reviews and presentation of information in these situations serve only to complete checklists and provide inappropriate feelings of accomplishment. Brief, meaningful encounters with the known noncompliant patients are necessary to check for new interest. In the value equation, unrealistic interventions render the equation out of balance with the lack of outcomes and overuse of scarce resources.

- Frequency of vital signs. When a patient has consistent and stable vital signs, is it still necessary to repeat these measures every four hours, especially since caregivers are present who can monitor the patient?
- Telemetry monitoring. Is all telemetry monitoring value based? Is the intervention of telemetry monitoring linked to outcomes that improve the patient's status and available resources?
- Searching for equipment. Does this task promote the patient's healing continuum?
- Searching for supplies. Is this an appropriate task for nurses?
- Passing out meal trays. Is this the best use of a nurse's time? Should someone from another division do this task?
- Searching for other providers and colleagues. Is this an appropriate task for nurses?
- Replenishing procedure carts; monitoring levels in supply rooms. Does this directly affect the patient?
- Searching for information and reference manuals. Can this be managed differently?

Improvements that focus on the elimination of non-valued-added work and increase productivity include computerized electronic health records, technology for communication, pocket reference guides, personal digital assistants, and pocket-sized hand sanitizer packets.

Elimination of non-value-added work provides time for nurses to comfort and talk with patients, develop and update plans of care, and provide patient and family education, which is work that is typically omitted when time is scarce.

Standardized Language

Another expectation is the use of standardized language in which the interventions of nursing must be specified and described with sufficient clarity that another researcher or practitioner can replicate the action. Standardized language comprises terminology and communication styles that can be used in all settings by all clinicians, is grounded in clinical practice and research, and is functionally appropriate for computerized clinical documentation systems to simplify the exchange, and makes it easier to manage and integrate clinical data into the electronic health record. The language must allow for the measurement of patient, family, and community health care interventions and outcomes (Moorhead et al., 2004).

Expected Nursing Outcomes

The evidence supporting a relationship between caregiver performance, patient outcomes, and financial performance is strong (Aiken, Smith, & Lake, 1994; Aiken, Clark, Cheung, Sloane, & Silber, 2003; Cho, Ketefian, Barkauskas, et al., 2003; Blegen & Vaughn, 1998; McCue, Mark, & Harless, 2003). Evidence of the relationships between variables in the organizational structure and patient outcomes has been also identified. Unfortunately, the intervening specific work processes that produce those outcomes have not been clearly articulated, nor are they embedded in the analysis of these relationships.

Once the work of nursing is described, the linkage to patient outcome and available resources must be established. The value equation in which there is an examination of clinical practice, performance outcomes, and the available payment structure serves as a template to assess overall value. The outcomes of nursing interventions include achievement of clinical goals, improvement in the ability to manage one's own health, and a safe environment as measured by the absence of adverse outcomes. Examples of outcomes specific to nursing that impact not only the patient, but the conditions that impact a patient's health include:

- Increased ability to provide self care
- Improved mobility
- Improved stress management and coping skills
- Improved knowledge of clinical condition
- Improved knowledge of healthy behaviors specific to nutrition and mobility
- Improved parenting skills
- Community health/well-being
- Improved knowledge of behaviors for safety specific to health care

Historically, health care leaders have believed that it is impossible to objectively quantify the clinical, social, and caring work of nursing in an aggregate manner and yet obtain objective and reliable data. However, quantifying and enumerating the work of nursing must be embraced to create valid and reliable information that will serve to increase the visibility and value of nursing within the health care environment, which in turn will provide credibility within the financial sectors of health care. Responding to this challenge is required for the advancement of the profession.

Computerized Nursing Information

Readily accessible information from powerful software including easy data input necessarily improves the consistent and standardized collection and measurement of patient information. Systems to support documentation of interventions, achievement of patient goals, the time and skill mix of caregivers required to achieve the goals, and examination of the relationship of these variables are essential. This documentation provides critical information to link the economic viability of the organization with resources, outcomes, and value-based service, satisfaction of nursing, and the performance of nursing using evidence-based interventions.

Context in Which Nursing Work Occurs

As discussed in Chapter 4, the impact of the work environment, or the conditions in which nursing care is provided, has a significant impact on patient outcomes. The information specific to the location, physical environment, organizational culture, operational structure, technology, and the availability of support services is necessary for determining the conditions in which nursing interventions are or are not effective. Pinkerton and Rivers (2001) identified 64 variables that impact nurse staffing needs, including variables specific to interdepartmental, intradepartmental, the care environment, professional competency, physicians, and the external environment. This nurse work complexity requires appropriate systems to assess and integrate measures of the multiple variables including actual nurse hours and context variables for a credible clinical productivity system. The following five major variables each contribute to the complexity of system processes and the achievement of desired outcomes: physical environment, organizational culture, organizational structure, technology, and support systems.

Physical Environment

A range of design characteristics—such as single versus double rooms, reduced noise, improved lighting, better ventilation, better ergonomic designs, workplaces that better support tasks, and improved layout—can reduce errors, reduce stress, improve sleep, reduce pain and drugs, and improve other outcomes. There is compelling scientific evidence from over 600 studies showing that design impacts staff and clinical outcomes (Ulrich et al., 2004). When the design supports clinical practice processes, patient healing in a stress-minimizing environment and worker productivity should increase dramatically.

Organizational Culture

Commitment to behaviors and values that support and expect shared leadership, nurse–physician collaboration, therapeutic relationships, and visible accountability for these behaviors positively impacts caregiver work processes.

Evidence continues to emerge supporting the relationships between behaviors and values of healing, and respect and accountability, with more efficient and effective processes (Neuhauser, 2002).

Operational Structure

The structure of the organization, namely, the decision-making processes, types of caregivers, skill mix percentages, and availability of expert resources such as hospitalists and advance practice nurses, clearly actualize the mission and vision of the organization as well as support the desired organizational culture and work of caregivers. Unit-based management tools to examine patient care quality, processes, outcomes, and costs are also essential operational tools that support first-time, effective decision-making in a timely manner.

Technology

The challenges of time and distance are disappearing with computer-enabled health care delivery and information that have been reconfigured to be available virtually everywhere (Ligon & Das, 2004). The availability of electronic, computerized, and integrated systems for patient care is believed to decrease the use of labor resources and increase the quality of organizational outcomes. Consideration must be given to the impact of the electronic health record, computerized physician order entry, physiologic monitoring, electronic medication administration records, scanning capabilities, and the integration of or lack of integration of these systems when determining the productivity measure. Wide variations in the availability of technology are found not only among organizations, but also among departments within each organization.

Support Systems

The presence of support systems for clinical caregivers directly impacts the ability of nurses to perform the work of nursing. These support systems include the availability of pharmacy, housekeeping, transportation, and messenger services 24 hours a day/seven days a week. The lack of or partial availability of support resources historically has resulted in nurses adding nonclinical tasks to their workload, thus decreasing clinical productivity. Table 8.2 summarizes the five categories of context variables.

Quantify the Work of Nursing in an Economic Model

The third step in creating a model for the future is to quantify the value-based work of nursing identified in the second step of the process. In addition,

Table 8.2   Aggregated Productivity Measurements of Context Variables

Physical Environment	Organizational Culture	Operational Structure	Technology	Support Systems
Single bed rooms	Shared leadership	Point-of-care decision making	Electronic health record, fully interfaced programs	Messenger
Noise control	Physician–nurse collaboration	Expert resources: Hospitalists/Advanced Practice Nurses	Computerized physician order entry	Transportation
Hand-washing dispensers	Values of respect, accountability, and healing	Decentralized pharmacists	Clinical documentation	Pharmacy
Patient lift system	Bilingual/ multilingual associates	Adequate staffing	Electronic medication administration record	
Medication preparation rooms	Community partnership	Management tools to evaluate work processes and outcomes	Scanning system	
Family space				
Ergonomic work stations		Patient classification system		
Adequate lighting & ventilation				

this quantification must consider the impact of the five contextual variables, that is, the physical environment, organizational culture, operational structure, technology, and support systems. The purpose of quantification is to develop information to extend the current productivity system that identifies the direct link between the evidence-based work of caregivers, patient outcomes, and payment. Necessarily, this requires quantification of (1) the specific work and (2) the link or relationship of the work to the achievement of desired patient outcomes. The health status of the patient must be positively impacted to justify resource expenditure.

The historical adequacy of the overarching position of medicine and its specific measures of procedural-based coding and billing has precluded the need for more accurate clinical productivity for nursing that is quantifiable, credible, and useful. Unfortunately, development of appropriate measures for nursing work only garners attention during times of nursing shortage and nursing dissatisfaction.

Organizations struggle to control costs through cost reductions of the poorly defined work of nursing, yet the need for competently educated practitioners continues to be significant. Despite the increases in nursing education and the increasing complexity of nursing work, clarity in the work of nursing and appropriate workload measures have not emerged to achieve the desired recognition of the value of nursing work in the marketplace. Poorly defined and described, uncertain nursing work is difficult to measure and evaluate, which too often results in uncertain patient outcomes. When attempts are made to decrease or increase nursing resources for work that is poorly defined, the impact on patient outcomes is uncertain as well. While it is believed that less nursing care results in poor patient outcomes, such conclusions are not universally supported. The lack of evidence identifying the specific interventions of nursing and their resulting impact on patient outcomes must be addressed. Simple hours of care without delineation of the actual work performed cannot be assuredly correlated to patient outcomes, whether they are positive or negative. Describing the work of nursing from an evidence-based perspective is the first step in the process; the second step, integrating these principles into practice, is evolutionary and ongoing.

These monitoring, integrating, and evaluating roles of nurses need to be captured adequately in a more appropriate clinical productivity system. The summative list of tasks based on the manufacturing model of work has not traditionally encompassed these processes. Clear and quantifiable information is needed that identifies the specific amount of nursing work performed by a specific level of caregiver, and the resulting quantifiable patient outcomes.

Aggregating Care for Quantification

The historical inadequacy of summative task workload calculations can be improved upon by using an aggregated or comprehensive workload unit approach to measure patient care that better represents the essence of the work of nursing. This comprehensive unit of service (CUS) captures the nonlinear nature of nursing practice, the routine multitasking, and frequent interruptions. A CUS is developed using expert opinion or expert panel methodology for determining workload time and skill mix standards. A panel of experts, individuals with a great deal of experience and the ability to estimate time in their area of expertise, identifies the time requirements. This consensus approach uses professional judgment to assess staff, which provides a flexible approach focused on a critical review of nursing practice, staffing, and the utilization of both supply and demand information (Dunn, Norby, Cournoyer, Hudec, O'Donnell, & Snider, 1995). Service work and one-of-a-kind jobs make setting time standards with more traditional techniques cost-prohibitive. Some workers never do the same thing twice. However, goals are needed. An expert is necessary to estimate every job and maintain a log of estimations. The "best estimation" technique is a low cost, fast, and initially acceptable way of quantifying information using estimation and self-reporting techniques. The "expert opinion" technique attempts to remedy the criticism of the inability of the work sampling technique to capture professional judgment required in health care (Dunn et al.). Since sampling can easily become biased and does not always reflect current conditions, it is only reliable if the results obtained approximate those results generated by experts.

In health care, the expert panel approach has been used to create a CUS as the foundational workload unit of measure for the Expert Nurse–Patient Classification System (Malloch & Conovoloff, 1999). Experienced nurses create workload standards from a comprehensive perspective of the work performed; expert nurses compile the nurse interventions provided to a patient for an entire shift or event, and identify the time required to provide this care as a unit rather than as summation of tasks. This approach integrates the multitasking processes of nurses and avoids the risk of double counting any tasks. Typically, the expert panel consists of nurses who practice in clinical, educational, research, and administrative roles such as experienced staff nurses, clinical nurse specialists, nurse managers, and associate nurse executives. The panel of nurses collaborates to estimate the amount of time and level of caregiver (skill mix) required to provide the total care in the CUS.

Consider the following care situation representing one shift of patient care. The patient is totally dependent for physical care, having difficulty communicating, unable to identify pain, hemodynamically unstable, and the Spanish-speaking family is having difficulty with the current full code status. An expert panel of nurses reviewed these care needs and determined the appropriate skill mix and hours of care needed as the standard for this type of care (Table 8.3). A total of 4.5 hours of care in a 12-hour shift were identified.

Table 8.3 Comprehensive Unit of Service: Complex Medical Patient

Category	Patient Needs	Caregiver Interventions
Cognitive Status	Responds to name by opening eyes— no verbalization other than garbled phrases.	Assess & monitor cog. Status q. 2 hrs.
Self-Care	Totally dependent.	Provide total ADLs, hygiene & mobility; requires 2 persons.
Emotional/Social/ Spiritual	Minimal social interaction.	Provide emotional support q. 6–8 hrs.
Comfort/Pain Management	Assess—but no indication of pain.	Assess & monitor non self-reporting pt. at least q. 6–8 hrs.
Family Information	Niece/spouse & others. Spanish-speaking, freq. visits.	Family conference re: code status. Requires q. 4–6 hour reinforcement of realistic expectations; Support through interpreter at least q. 2 hrs.
Treatments & Interventions	Hemodynamically unstable (mod.) Respiratory failure Full code.	Dialysis, meds—IVP & IVPB q. 2 hrs. Monitor ventilator status q. 15 minutes; Titrate 3 drips; provide trach care × 2
Interdisciplinary Coordination/Patient Teaching and Documentation	Change in code status.	Freq. communication with > 4 services.
Transition Needs	Pt. not meeting goals.	Plan for family conference. Modify care plan.
EXPERT TIME ESTIMATION	Total Hrs. (12 Hr. Shift): 4.5	RN 2.5 LPN/LVN .5 NA 1.5

Standardized Patient Classification Systems

Quantifying the work of nursing using a standardized approach to patient acuity is the foundation for a valid and reliable patient classification system, another important element of an evidence-based workload management system. The patient classification used by an organization must reflect the major clinical intervention categories applicable to all clinical specialties. At a minimum, categories specific to the technical work of nursing, monitoring activities, interdisciplinary coordination, communication, and leadership must be represented.

The nonreducible CUS, rather than the single task, as the unit of workload measurement better represents the work of nursing. Consistency in the description and quantification of caregiver interventions using the CUS is the foundational unit for a valid and reliable clinical productivity management system. Further, computerization of the collection and management of these data supports reduced variability and subjectivity in patient classification systems historically fraught with inconsistency and mistrust.

Multidisciplinary Units of Service

Extension of the nursing patient classification system to include all disciplines providing care further advances the robustness of a clinical productivity system. The ideal workload management system is one in which the unit of service is multidisciplinary and patient-specific for a defined period of time. All disciplines providing services are integrated and considered as a "multidisciplinary comprehensive unit of service (MCUS)." The work of each discipline can be identified on the basis of interventions and associated contributions to patient outcomes. The MCUS represents the integrated, interwoven contributions of associated disciplines such as physical therapy, respiratory therapy, and social services. An example of a MCUS is provided in Table 8.4, which illustrates the quantification of patient care for all contributing disciplines within a defined period of time. In this exemplar, the interventions of social workers and respiratory and physical therapists are integrated into workflow and processes along with the registered nurse (RN), licensed practical nurse, and nursing assistants. Using the expert panel method, experts determined that a total of 6.5 hours of care for all six disciplines was necessary. The appropriate percentage of the six disciplines is also identified.

New Approach to Clinical Productivity

In a study on hospital nurse productivity, Eastaugh (2002) analyzed the impact of the current trend toward using nurse extenders or unlicensed personnel.

Table 8.4   Multidisciplinary Comprehensive Unit of Service: Complex Medical Patient

Category	Patient Needs	Caregiver Interventions
Cognitive Status	Responds to name by opening eyes—no verbalization other than garbled phrases.	Assess & monitor cog. Status q. 2 hrs.
Self-Care	Totally dependent	Provide total ADLs, hygiene & mobility; requires 2 persons. Physical therapist assistance with range of motion.
Emotional/Social/Spiritual	Minimal social interaction.	Provide emotional support q. 6–8 hrs.
Comfort/Pain Management	Assess—but no indication of pain.	Assess & monitor non self-reporting pt. at least q. 6–8 hrs.
Family Information	Niece/spouse & others. Spanish-speaking, freq. visits.	Family conference re: code status. Requires q. 4–6 hour reinforcement of realistic expectations; Support through interpreter at least q. 2 hrs.
Treatments & Interventions	Hemodynamically unstable (mod.) Respiratory failure Full code.	Dialysis, meds—IVP & IVPB q. 2 hrs. Monitor ventilator status q. 15 minutes; Titrate 3 drips; provide trach care × 2; respiratory therapy management of ventilator.
Interdisciplinary Coordination/Patient Teaching and Documentation	Change in code status.	Freq. communication with > 4 services. Social worker communication > 1 hr.
Transition Needs	Pt. not meeting goals.	Plan for family conference. Modify care plan.
EXPERT TIME ESTIMATION	**Total Hrs. (12 Hr. Shift): 6.5 hours**	**RN 2.5** **Social Worker 1.25** **LPN 0.5** **Physical Therapist 0.25** **NA 1.5** **Respiratory Therapist 0.50**

Data from 37 hospitals using primary nursing, all RN staff, and team nursing were compared, and the study concluded that the tradition of 100% RN primary care nursing must be abandoned, given that it was the least productive and not affordable with the current funding limitations. A significant omission noted in this analysis, however, was that there was no mention or analysis of output or the patient outcomes specific to each delivery model. While the use of RNs' hours was the highest in the all-RN delivery model, more information is needed before such a broad conclusion can be drawn. It is possible that the overall long-term cost of this model is the most economical due to the absence of nosocomial infections, patient falls, and medication errors.

Historically, the measurement of productivity has remained a reflection of resources used compared to budgeted resources or hours used for each patient unit of service without considering the specific work performed to achieve the results. The importance and significance of knowing which outcomes resulted from which work performed by which category of caregiver are critically necessary in order for the profession to advance the articulation of its value and contribution to the health of individuals. Understanding these important relationships between specific work processes and integrating them into the productivity measurement systems of organizations requires new knowledge, new mental models, and commitment to staffing on the basis of evidence or the trend data created from best practices.

Unfortunately, this approach and limited analysis have been used in most organizations to measure nurse productivity and to make significant decisions specific to the allocation of staffing resources. The hours used are compared to patient unit of service without consideration of the actual output, which is an essential component of a productivity measure. These traditional productivity measures of "hours used per patient day" represent a limited analysis and do not reflect the notion of theoretical productivity, which calls for the greatest output for the least input (Drucker, 1990).

Measurements that are limited to total hours worked per patient day comparisons to projected budgeted hours can only serve the financial analyst. Such comparisons provide no information specific to the level of patient acuity, provision of appropriate interventions, achievement of clinical outcomes, and absence of adverse outcomes, all of which require a framework for productivity measurement based on principles that integrate values of effectiveness, utility, and cost. Productivity measurement that reflects and supports the position and complex production involved in the practice of nursing, rather than the functional efficiency comparison of hours worked to hours budgeted, is needed. Metrics that reflect the output of care compared to the input of providers and adjusted for environmental factors, provide a more accurate representation of nursing productivity.

Embed the Framework for Aggregated, Adjusted Productivity Measurement Within Existing Systems

The fourth consideration addresses the need for an aggregated productivity measurement that encompasses a combination of inputs and outputs, and is expressed and examined in a matrix format rather than a single productivity ratio calculation of output to input. Current measurement and payment systems, while cumbersome and outdated, can serve as vehicles to create improved systems. Any consideration for modifications to existing systems should emphasize the need to improve the value of data and their utility to the health care system. Consistency of definitions, attribution of value to work processes specific to the mission of the organization and patient clinical status, and reimbursement specific to value rather than procedures performed should also drive any modifications.

The current metric of hours per patient day identifies how long it took for the care, but not what was done; it is an incomplete representation of the work of nursing (simplicity) that does not incorporate structural and environment considerations in productivity measures. Relative value unit (RVU) measures attempt to recognize the degree of patient care variation based on a median unit but are limited by the description of the value of 1.0 unit. The limited accuracy and completeness of describing the 1.0 RVU continues to be problematic because descriptors for all categories of the core work of nursing are not included.

The purpose of modifying current processes and measures is not to devalue the historical clinical productivity measurement, but rather to extend the existing productivity system to quantify the relationship between patient care services, value, and payment, and to adjust for the variables impacting the work of nursing. The Medicare payment system, International Classification of Diseases codes, and other accepted billing and reimbursement models can be strengthened with additional principles and parameters. To be sure, this work is not without challenge. Re-engineering anything is a risk that requires knowledge of not only the desired state of improvement, but also of failures that one desires to correct. Successes provide confidence that something right is occurring, but not necessarily why it is right. Failures provide unquestionable proof that we have done something wrong. Creating new models for health care clinical labor productivity requires knowledge of the best features of effective existing processes and failures that have negatively impacted outcomes (Table 8.5).

Evaluate the Results

The fifth consideration is evaluation. As previously noted, the financial representation of nursing's throughput or interventions is best determined using the value equation consisting of a combination of quality, cost-effectiveness, and service. The value equation now serves as the vital unifier and clarifying

Table 8.5   Clinical Productivity Evaluation Matrix

Input Caregivers *hours of care/ skill mix*	Input Caregiver *actual interventions*	Required hours of care *patient acuity/ variance*	Context *variables/ adjustments*	Output *patient clinical outcomes*	Output *patient safety outcomes*
RN	Assess & monitor	Plus or minus 5% comparing actual to patient classification needs.	Physical Environment	Respiratory stability	Falls
LPN	Administer medications		Organizational Culture	Knowledge of disease	Medication errors
NA	Insert IV line		Operational Structure	Minimal medications	Nosocomial infections
Critical Thinking	Patient education		Technology	Patient satisfaction	Medical errors
Certification	Assess/monitor		Support Systems		
Advanced Practice Nurses	Family education/ support				
Technicians	Coordinate care				
	Document care				

link between service and cost (Malloch & Porter-O'Grady, 1999). All care providers must now know the relationship between what they do, what it costs, and what is achieved as a result of having done it. But the challenge remains to determine a good number for clinical productivity. Is there a single metric that is robust enough to reflect clinical productivity? If so, what is the number?

The continuing dilemma to have adequate RN surveillance and yet remain cost effective begs the question as to what the ideal number of nurses per patient and the mix of caregivers should be for a given group of patients. Inadequate numbers of RNs lead to "failure to rescue" situations, and total RN staffing is not required for all types of patient care. The answer lies somewhere in between.

While adequate numbers of nurses are essential to avoid "failure to rescue" situations, specific patient information is needed to determine safe staffing. To be sure, as long as patients vary, the ratio of patients assigned to nurses will vary. But it is more than the right number or ratio of nurses; it is the right nurse doing the right things during the time available. Staffing ratios in which nurses are performing clerical services, finding equipment, and low-skill clinical activities seriously undermine the perceptions of staffing adequacy. To date, the ideal ratio of nurses to patients has not been identified; rather, a range of numbers of patients has been hypothesized for specific clinical areas (Curtin, 2003).

One hundred percent productivity requires homogeneity, that is, patients with the same disease, patients arriving at the same rate, providers equal in their ability to provide patient care, and families with the same level of knowledge and understanding. The most reasonable approach for operational decision-making is longitudinal monitoring of productivity by organizational units combined with indicators of quality of patient care (O'Brien-Pallas et al., 2004). This care must be described, documented, and measured using a standardized patient classification system to support decisions that will support safe patient care.

O'Brien-Pallas and colleagues identified 85% (± 5%) as the optimal nursing unit productivity with 93% as the maximum productivity because 7% of the shift is made up of mandatory breaks.

Data analysis of nursing work using the best available evidence is an expected standard of practice. Several methods of economic evaluation are available for consideration. Each method is based on specific goals (Stone, Curran, & Bakken, 2002) and includes the following:

- Cost minimization: Costs are compared between alternatives only. Equal effects are assumed. No outcomes are measured.
- Cost-effectiveness: Consequences are measured in the same units between alternatives. Outcomes are measured using ratios such as $/outcome or $/life year gained.

- Cost utility: Effects include both quantity and quality measures. Measures are dollars of quality of life years gained.
- Cost benefit: Effects are measured as a single dollar measure. Measures are in dollars gained.
- Cost consequences: Costs and effects are listed separately. Effects between alternatives may have different measures. Dollars and a separate list of outcomes are measured.

Each of these evaluation methods offers a different lens from which to examine the work of nursing. A combination of several methods better represents nursing work based on the intended goals and resources.

Variance Management

The sixth and final consideration in the clinical productivity model of the future is variance management. The most significant information produced from any system is that specific to the variances or differences between the desired and the actual. Seldom is there a perfect match between what is desired and the actual results. The resulting variance between needs and resources is a reality of workload processes with the inherent expectations for reducing, eliminating, or managing these differences. It is this variance that provides the data from which to manage, monitor, and improve system performance. Merely counting and documenting the desired and actual does not provide any value for the system in outcome management. Accountability for the articulation and reporting of variance management is an essential unifying link in the process. Producing high levels of quality without human or financial resources is irrational and doomed to eliminate (destroy) the system. Effective evaluation processes lay the foundation for safe and timely management of the variance between what is desired and what actually occurs.

Leaders are continually challenged to consider variations in the known natural clinical variances of disease, levels of severity, patients' responses to treatment, variability in work flow due to random arrivals of patients, and the inherent variability of clinicians specific to knowledge, critical thinking, prioritizing, and communication. According to Long (2002), the goal is to eliminate "artificial variance," the clinical errors, medication errors, lack of knowledge, inappropriate scheduling, and scheduling based on staff needs rather than patient needs. Leaders should focus on managing the natural variation or the uncertain occurrence of care needs by patients, both predicted and unpredicted, and the inherent professional differences in ability. "System variances" result in high and low levels of work-load, and frequent internal diversion of patients to other units, back-ups in the post-anesthesia care unit, external diversion from the emergency department, staff overload, and increased length of stay from the system gridlock. When a system variance is identified, the following management practices are appropriate:

1. Delineate protocols and link their required interventions to desired outcomes
2. Create a framework to examine performance standards
3. Define the linkage between interventions, best practice, and payment formats
4. Continue to monitor, evaluate, and adjust for gaps in desired linkages needed for value (cost-service-quality)

A "staffing variance" occurs when there is a difference between the identified patient care needs and the available resources to meet those needs. Given that there will always be discrepancies between needs and available staff, and given that nurses will continue to accept responsibility for providing safe, competent care, strategies to manage the variance are essential. When a staffing variance is identified, and efforts to obtain additional staff are exhausted, consider the following 10 strategies:

1. Teamwork: Commit to working as a team to address the gap. Planned variance management from a team perspective is proactive and stress-minimizing. Individual variance management is impulsive, reactive, and highly stressful.
2. Prioritize: Identify specific patient care issues that require immediate attention and those that can be safely left until later in the shift or for the next shift.
3. Decision-making: As a team, determine how work will be organized or reorganized, and then assign work for the shift based on the type of staff available and patient needs. Decide which aspects of care can be eliminated or safely assigned to others.
4. Delegate and supervise: Delegate work to the appropriate caregivers and supervise accordingly to ensure that the work is being performed as required.
5. Control workflow to the unit. Reroute admissions if possible and appropriate.
6. Communicate: Arrange for a short report mid-shift to assess how well all team members are managing the workload, and re-assign and reprioritize as needed. Communicate how breaks and lunches will be organized.
7. Plan: Once the team is organized, have each team member do a quick walkabout to assess those clients identified as high-priority.
8. Evaluate: If circumstances require modification of patient's plan of care, inform patients about changes in their respective plan of care and provide clear factual information to patients about the care they can expect.

9. Document: Complete a variance report that identifies the specific patient care concerns. Clearly describe the safety concerns. Provide examples of care that could not be completed or what prescribed frequencies for interventions were delayed.

10. Communicate: Share the variance management data with stakeholders and develop plans to minimize future gaps.

Obstacles to a New Productivity Management System

Despite clear and convincing theoretical rationale for system change, the obstacles to making it happen cannot be ignored or taken lightly. Creating a new model for productivity measurement and management requires support, passion, and resources. For many health care leaders, making a significant system change is far too complex to embrace. Many leaders will struggle with any modification of the current system under the misguided notions that the system is functional and provides the appropriate information to make decisions supportive of quality patient care outcomes. The control and influence of the current powerful organizational infrastructure over nursing resource allocation, coupled with the inability of nursing to articulate its specific work and outcomes achieved within the existing productivity framework, are difficult for many to challenge.

Simplicity

The simplicity of ratio calculations of two variables has overshadowed the multiple data values needed for accuracy. Overcoming the deeply entrenched tradition of ratio- or grid-based staffing models to create evidence-based processes that recognize and address the daily variations of patient care needs and staff availability requires courage and commitment to the creation of a better system. The obvious simplicity of these historical calculations is antithetical to the real goal of quality patient care. To overcome this resistance, increasing numbers of organizations are selecting computerized database management systems to provide more sophisticated, more complex, and timelier data that can be used to develop the next generation of productivity measurement. The reality is that it is difficult to use resources effectively without such systems and evaluations.

The "moral dilemmas" associated with variance management, namely, prioritizing work and/or delaying nurse work, are difficult to accept. Coupled with the historical nursing emphasis on the social mandate for care and positive perception of the public, nurses are further reluctant as individuals to not attempt to do as much as possible. The long-embedded nursing behaviors of oppression, dominance of the medical model, and fluctuating supply of nurses have discouraged nurses from challenging the system. Not only are new models of productivity needed, but also new skills for nurses to understand and practice in an environment based on evidence and value.

SUMMARY

A new clinical productivity system will serve to decrease or minimize current practices specific to the management of nursing resources, which ultimately impact the viability of the organization providing health care services. Altering the response to nurse resource shortages in a manner that advances the economic, social, and political state of nursing requires new thinking. Efforts to increase or decrease the number and skills of nurses can be sustained only with evidence specific to support the structure, processes, and expected outcomes of nursing. If not, the cyclical shortages will continue with resulting frustration and expectations for future recurrence. According to Gilenas and Loh (2004), there is not a lack of knowledge linking work force and quality; rather, there is a performance gap because of the lack of execution. Using an evidence-based approach to clinical productivity management presents nursing with a significant but essential challenge, a challenge that today's nurses are well suited to address.

REFERENCES

Aiken, L. H., Clark, S. P., Cheung, R. B., Sloane, D. M., & Silber, J. H. (2003). Education levels of hospital nurses and patient mortality. *Journal of the American Medical Association, 290*(12), 1–8.

Aiken, L. H., Clark, S. P., Sloane, D. M., Sochalski J., & Silber, J. H. (2002). Hospital nurse staffing and patient mortality, nurse burnout, and job dissatisfaction. *Journal of the American Medical Association, 288*(16), 1987–1993.

Aiken, L. H., Smith, H. L., & Lake, E. T. (1994). Lower Medicare mortality among a set of hospitals known for good nursing care. *Medical Care, 32*(8), 771–787.

American Nurses Association. (2000). *Nurse Staffing and Patient Outcomes in the Inpatient Hospital Setting.* Washington, DC: American Nurses Publishing.

American Nurses Association. (2003). *Nursing's Social Policy Statement,* 2nd ed. Washington, DC: American Nurses Publishing.

Ashley, J. A. (1976). *Hospitals, Paternalism, and the Role of the Nurse.* New York, NY: Teachers College Press.

Barry-Walker, J. (2000). The impact of assistance redesign on staff, patients, and financial outcomes. *Journal of Nursing Administration, 30*(2), 77–89.

Berry, L., Parker, D., Coile, R., Hamilton, K., O'Neill, D., & Sadler, B. (2004). *Can Better Buildings Improve Care and Increase Your Financial Returns?* Chicago, IL: Frontiers of Health Services Management.

Blegen, M. A., & Vaughn, T. (1998). A multisite study of nurse staffing and patient occurrences. *Nursing Economic$, 16*(4), 196–203.

Buerhaus, P. (1995). Economics and reform: Forces affecting nurse staffing. *Nursing Policy Forum, 1*(2), 8–14.

Buerhaus, P., & Needleman, J. (2000). Policy implication of research on nurse staffing and quality of care. *Policy, Politics & Nursing Practice, 1*(1), 5–16.

Buerhaus, P. (1991). Dynamic shortage of registered nurses. *Nursing Economic$, 9*(5), 371–328.

Butterworth, V. (1979). *Girls in White.* Independence, MO: Herald Publishing House.

Child, A. P., Institute of Medicine (U.S.), Board on Health Care Services, Committee on the Work Environment for Nurses and Patient Safety, & NetLibrary Inc. (2004). *Keeping Patients Safe: Transforming the Work Environment of Nurses.* Washington, DC: National Academies Press.

Cho, S. H., Ketefian, S., Barkauskas, V. H., et al. (2003). The effect of nurse staffing on adverse outcomes, morbidity, mortality and medical costs. *Nursing Research, 52*(2), 71–79.

Corey, M. (2001). *Groups: Process and Practice.* London, UK: Wadsworth Publishing.

Curtin, L. (2003, September). An integrated analysis of nurse staffing and related variables: Effects on patient outcomes. *Online Journal of Issues in Nursing.* Available at http://www.nursingworld.org/ojin/topic22/tpc22_5.htm. Retrieved March 2005.

Duffy, W. (2004). Representing our value. *AORN Journal, 80*(2), 197–200.

Drucker, P. (1990). *Managing the Nonprofit Organization.* New York, NY: Harper Collins.

Dunn, M. G., Norby, R., Cournoyer, P., Hudec, S., O'Donnell, J., & Snider, M. D. (1995). Expert panel method for nurse staffing and resource management. *Journal of Nursing Administration, 25*(10), 61–67.

Eastaugh, S. (1998). *Healthcare Finance: Costs, Productivity, and Strategic Design.* Boston, MA: Jones and Bartlett.

Eastaugh, S. R. (2002). Hospital nurse productivity. *Journal of Health Care Finance, 29*(1), 14–22.

Eberhardt, B. J., Szigeti, E., & University of North Dakota, Bureau of Business and Economic Research. (1990). Predictors of nursing staff turnover intentions in North Dakota nursing homes: Implications for management practice. Grand Forks, ND: University of North Dakota Press.

Faass, N. (2001). *Integrating Complementary Medicine into Health Systems.* Gaithersburg, MD: Aspen Publishers.

Finkler, S., & Graf, C. (2001). *Budgeting Concepts for Nurse Managers.* New York, NY: W. B. Saunders.

Gilenas, L., & Loh, D. Y. (2004). The effect of workforce issues on patient safety. *Nursing Economic$, 22*(5), 266–272, 279.

Harrington, C., & Estes, C. L. (2004). *Health Policy: Crisis and Reform in the U.S. Health Care Delivery System,* 4th ed. Sudbury, MA: Jones and Bartlett.

Hope, H. (2004). Working conditions of the nursing workforce: Excerpts from a policy roundtable at academy house 2003 annual research meeting. *Health Service Research, 39*(3), 445–455.

Horak, B., Welton, W., & Shortell, S. (2004). Crossing the quality chasm: Implications for health services administration education. *Journal of Health Administration Education, 21*(1), 15–38.

Hughes, E. C., & American Nurses Association. (1958). *Twenty Thousand Nurses Tell Their Story; A Report on Studies of Nursing Functions Sponsored by the American Nurses Association.* Philadelphia, PA: Lippincott.

Institute of Medicine (U.S.). Committee on Quality of Health Care in America. & NetLibrary Inc. (2001). *Crossing the Quality Chasm: A New Health System for the 21st Century.* Washington, DC: National Academy Press.

Johnson C. (2002). How busy are you? *Harvard Business Review, 80*(10), 132.

Kalisch, P., & Kalisch, B. (2003). *American Nursing: A History.* Philadelphia, PA: Lippincott Williams & Wilkins.

King, C. R., & Hinds, P. S. (2003). *Quality of Life: From Nursing and Patient Perspectives: Theory, Research, Practice* (2nd ed.). Sudbury, MA: Jones and Bartlett.

Lanser, E. G. (2001). Leveraging your nursing resources. *Healthcare Executive, 80*(10), 50–51.

Ligon, K., & Das, E. (2004, October). The benefits of automated nursing documentation. *Nurse Leader,* 29–31.

Long, M. C. (2002). *Translating the Principles of Variability Management into Reality: One Physician's Perspective.* Boston, MA: Boston University: School of Management, Executive Learning.

Malloch, K., & Conovoloff, A. J. (1999). Patient Classification Systems, Part 1: The third generation. *JONA, 29*(7/8), 49–56.

Malloch, K., & Porter-O'Grady, T. (1999). Partnership economics: Nursing's challenge in a quantum age. *Nursing Economic$, 17*(6), 299–307.

McCue, M., Mark, B. A., & Harless, D. W. (2003). Nurse staffing, quality, and financial performance. *Journal of Health Care Finance, 29*(4), 54–76.

Merriam-Webster's Collegiate Dictionary, 11th ed. (2002). Springfield, MA: Merriam-Webster, Inc.

Meyers, F. E., & Stewart, J. R. (2002). *Motion and Time Study for Lean Manufacturing,* 3rd ed. Upper Saddle River, NJ: Prentice Hall.

Moody, R. (2004). Nurse productivity measures for the 21st-century. *Healthcare Management Review, 29*(2), 98–106.

Moorhead, S., Johnson, M., & Maas, M. (2004). *Nursing Outcomes Classification (NOC),* 3rd ed. St. Louis, MO: C.V. Mosby.

Murphy, M. (2003). Research brief: Eliminating wasteful work in hospitals improves margin, quality, and culture. Washington, DC: Murphy Leadership Institute.

Needleman, J., Buerhaus, P., Mattke, S., et al. (2002). Nurse-staffing levels and the quality of care in hospitals. *New England Journal of Medicine, 346*(22), 1715–1722.

Neuhauser, P. C. (2002). Building a high-retention culture in healthcare: Fifteen ways to get good people to stay. *Journal of Nursing Administration, 32*(9), 470–478.

O'Brien-Pallas, L., Thomson, D., Hall, L. M., Pink, G., Kerr, M., Li, S. X., & Meyer, R. (2004). *Evidence-Based Standards for Measuring Nurse Staffing and Performance.* Available at http://www.chsrf. ca/final_research/ogc/obrien_e.php. Retrieved March 2005.

Pinkerton, S., & Rivers, R. (2001). Factors influencing staffing needs. *Nursing Economic$, 19*(5), 236–237.

Rice, V. H. (2000). *Handbook of Stress, Coping, and Health: Implications for Nursing Research, Theory, and Practice.* Thousand Oaks, CA: Sage.

Rubin, I. M., Plovnick, M. S., & Fry, R. E. (1975). *Improving the Coordination of Care: A Program for Health Team Development.* Cambridge, MA: Ballinger.

Smith, J. (2002). Analysis of differences in entry-level or and practice by educational preparation. *Journal of Nursing Education, 41*(11), 491–495.

Squires, A. (2004). A dimensional analysis of role enactment of acute care nurses. *Journal of Nursing Scholarship, 36*(3), 272–278.

Starr, P. (1984). *Social Transformation of American Medicine: The Rise of a Sovereign Profession in the Making of the Vast Industry.* New York, NY: Basic Books.

Stone, P. W., Curran, C. R., & Bakken, S. (2002). Economic evidence for evidence-based practice. *Journal of Nursing Scholarship, 34*(3), 277–282.

Traynor, M. (1999). *Managerialism and Nursing: Beyond Oppression and Profession.* London, UK: Rutledge Press.

Ulrich, R., Quan, X., Zimring, C., Joseph, A., & Choudhary, R. (2004). *The Role of the Physical Environment in the Hospital of the 21st Century: A Once-in-a-Lifetime Opportunity.* Concord, CA: Center for Health Design.

Waldman, J., Kelly, F., Arora, S., & Smith, H. (2004). The shocking cost of turnover in healthcare. *Healthcare Management Review, 29*(1), 2–7.

Wannisky, K. E., Centers for Medicare and Medicaid Services (U.S.), & United States. General Accounting Office. (2003). *Department of Health and Human Services, Centers for Medicare and Medicaid Services Medicare Program: Prospective Payment System and Consolidated Billing for Skilled Nursing Facilities—Update.* Available at http://purl.access.gpo.gov/GPO/LPS37825. Retrieved March 2005.

Weinberg, D. B., & Suzanne, G. (2004). *Code Green: Money-Driven Hospitals and the Dismantling of Nursing (The Culture and Politics of Healthcare Work).* New York, NY: Cornell University Press.

While, A., Forbes, A., Ullman, R., Lewis, S., Mathes, L., & Grifiths, P. (2004). Good practices that address continuity during transition from child to adult care: Synthesis of the evidence. *Childcare Health and Development, 30*(5), 439–452.

Whittmann-Price, R. (2004). Emancipation in decision-making in women's health. *Journal of Advanced Nursing, 47*(4), 437–445.

CHAPTER 9

Evidence-Based Practice and Health Policy: A Match or a Mismatch?

Susan R. Cooper, Virginia Trotter Betts, Karen Butler, and Jill Gentry

The emergence of evidence-based practice (EBP) as a popular process to promote informed health care delivery over the course of the past two decades has prompted health professionals, policy-makers, and the public to seriously consider if health policy should and could be informed by clinical EBPs. It has been suggested that evidence-based health policy would then be a next step and policy-makers should perhaps join this clinical bandwagon. However, a move to evidence-based health policy as a "best practice" will lead policy-makers to face some of the very same challenges, competing agendas, and shifting priorities that are present in the move to EBPs as a clinical norm. The aim of this chapter is to explore the relationship between EBP and health policy, and to identify some of the challenges, pro and con arguments, potential outcomes, and difficulties in drawing EBPs closer to health policy.

To understand the relationship between EBP and health policy, it is important to define some terminology. Policy is a purposeful plan of action aimed toward solving a problem or issue of concern in the public or private sector (Sudduth, 1999). Policy is both an entity and a process. As an entity, policy may be viewed as the "standing decisions" of an organization (Eulau & Prewitt, 1973) and often refers to goals, programs, and proposals (Milstead, 1999). Policy can be an action or nonaction, and is made in different venues including the legislative, judicial, and executive arenas, and/or within organizations both large and small. Policy is often the outcome of a complex labyrinth of decisions that develop over time as a result of competing agendas and necessary compromise.

Policy is a process when its stages are viewed over time. For governmental policy-making, these stages include agenda setting, legislation, and subsequent rule-making, program implementation, and program evaluation. The process involves a series of activities that brings an issue or problem to the government and results in direct action by the government to address the problem (Milio, 1989). Governmental policy-making occurs in a political environment (i.e., decisions about who gets what; when they get it; and how much they get) and is made within a context of power and influence, negotiation, and bargaining (Lasswell, 1958). Public policy directs problems to the government for a response (Jones, 1984). Public policy is generally developed by a governmental body or agency, but the use of evidence is also applicable to policy-making that occurs in the private sector and on an individualized level, that is, health care settings, professional organizations, a specific patient population by diagnosis, or all the citizens in a country (DePalma, 2004).

Health policy directly addresses health problems (Milstead, 1999). Health policy is generally classified using the determinants of health over which it is possible to have influence; these include the physical, biological, or social environment or health care services (Gray, 2001). There are two major reasons for health policy: (1) to change the way in which health care services are funded, organized, or held accountable (health care policies); and (2) to improve health through changes in the physical, biological, or social environments (health or public health policies) (Gray). Health care policies aim to improve efficiency, quality, accountability, or acceptability. Health or public health policies can impact the incidence and/or prevalence of disease (Gray).

While there is little disagreement that clinical decisions for an individual should be based upon the best available evidence, policy-makers are often faced with competing definitions of evidence in the health care field for policy purposes. Does the best evidence come only from randomized controlled trials or can the evidence come from observational studies? Certainly, even within health care clinical interactions, there is disagreement about what constitutes the best available evidence and/or an EBP.

EBP has evolved over the past two decades as an outgrowth of the rapid expansion of science and knowledge as well as innovative technology that increases the availability of research findings and the development of enhanced research methodologies. As these advances have been used to inform and support new practices, clinical decision-making has increasingly been based on research. This is the premise of evidence-based health care (Gray, 2001). Yet, others have defined EBP through other lenses, and definitions are variable and not always straightforward (Jennings & Loan, 2001).

The original definition pertaining specifically to evidence-based medicine (EBM) came from the predominately Canadian formed Evidence-Based Medicine Working Group (EBMWG):

Evidence-based medicine de-emphasizes intuition, unsystematic clinical experience, and pathophysiologic rationale as sufficient grounds for clinical decision making and stresses the examination of evidence from clinical research (EBMWG, 1992, p. 2420).

This definition emphasizes clinical research while giving less value to intuition and the clinical experience of health professionals. Rosenberg and Donald (1995) defined EBM as "the process of systematically finding, appraising and using contemporaneous research findings as the basis for clinical decisions" (p. 1222).

Sackett and colleagues (whose work is cited throughout many of the chapters in this text) expanded these definitions to include the "conscientious, explicit and judicious use of current best evidence in making decisions about the care of individual patients" (Sackett, Rosenberg, Gray, Haynes, & Richardson, 1996, p. 71). These authors went on to say that EBP involves using individual clinical expertise along with the best available external clinical evidence from systematic research. This definition is important for nurses in that it allows for clinical expertise as a building block of evidence while still emphasizing randomized controlled trials in the hierarchy of evidence (Jennings & Loan, 2001).

Definitions of EBP are found in nursing literature as well, and all emphasize evidence from research as a part of the fundamental definition. Gerrish and Clayton's (1998) definition of EBP emphasizes the use of research findings primarily from clinical trials or other types of experimental designs to evaluate nursing interventions. Stevens and Paugh (1999) seem to agree and propose a definition: "Evidence-based nursing [is] practice that relies on information generated from results of scientific research" (p. 155).

Goode and Piedalue (1999) expanded upon this definition to include other forms of evidence, such as pathophysiology, quality improvement and risk data, standards of care, infection control data, cost-effectiveness analysis, and benchmarking data. Perhaps the most significant differential in their definition was the addition of patient preference and nursing clinical expertise as forms of evidence to be used in the decision-making process. Accordingly, Ingersoll (2000) included the use of theory and research and acknowledged the value of the individual's needs and preferences in the delivery of evidence-based care.

Despite the varying definitions of EBP, all are intended to be used as models for establishing best practice. However, this inconsistency of definition, even in the familiar clinical context for which it was intended (i.e., the kind of evidence allowed, the value or weight of the evidence, and/or how that evidence should be utilized in decision-making), creates enormous difficulty for policy-makers because they may or (usually) may not have any experience in health care or research and are being asked to consider and/or apply EBP in the policy context.

LEVELING OR GRADING THE EVIDENCE

In addition to the multiplicity of definitions of evidence and various opinions about what constitutes best evidence, there are many published schemas available that can be used to grade evidence. The Agency for Healthcare Research and Quality (AHRQ) supported the publication of a guide to systems used to rate the strength of scientific evidence (West, King, Carey, Lohr, McKoy, Sutton, & Lux, 2002). The authors of this AHRQ study examined 121 systems designed to rate the strength of scientific evidence. The goals of this project were to "describe systems used to rate the strength of scientific evidence, including evaluating the quality of individual articles that make up a body of evidence on a specific scientific question in health care, and to provide some guidance as to 'best practices' in this field today" (p. 1).

Central to the discussion of evidence, of course, is the concept of quality. Methodological quality has been defined as "the extent to which all aspects of a study's design and conduct can be shown to protect against systemic bias, nonsystemic bias, and inferential error" (Lohr & Carey, 1999 as cited in West et al., 2002, p. 1). Gaps were identified in the AHRQ study in rating quality, strength of evidence, and application of grading schemas to "less traditional" bodies of evidence such as observational studies. Thus, these gaps may be of particular importance to nurses who are interested in defining evidence.

It is clear from the summary in the AHRQ work that there is not (nor is there likely to be in the near future) a single schema that can be used to grade evidence across all types of scholarly work. In addition, the evidence-gathering process will differ from clinician to clinician, researcher to researcher. These facts alone illustrate the problem of trying to determine exactly what evidence is and how it might be best applied in the policy process.

GETTING TO EVIDENCE-BASED HEALTH POLICY

Obstacles in the Search for Evidence

Even if policy-makers were determined to utilize evidence upon which to base their decisions in health care policy development, they would encounter formidable stumbling blocks along the way. Gray (2001) identifies these blocks as gaps and has suggested actions that can be taken to overcome them. Gaps identified include relevance, publication, hunting, and quality.

Relevance Gap

The relevance gap equates to the absence of high quality data that may exist, especially in certain conditions or situations. According to Gray, the research agenda is frequently dependent on investment in research and development. There are many areas without sufficient investments. The absence of high quality data in a particular area of health does not make decision-making impossible, but instead requires the use of the best available evidence using a well-researched published grading schema (Gray, 2001).

Publication Gap

The publication gap exists because, although the main source of evidence is in the published literature, not all evidence is published in scientific journals (Gray, 2001). Reasons cited for this gap include: researchers who fail to write up and submit their findings for publication; those who do not complete and submit for publication due to negative research results (submission bias); reluctance on the part of proprietary companies, such as pharmaceuticals, to publish information that may not show their products in the most advantageous light; biased editors who are more prone to publish positive rather than negative results (publication bias); and the influence of language because positive findings are more likely to be published in English language journals and negative findings in other language journals (language bias). Searching for unpublished data if time allows, or at least a thorough systematic review and conscious awareness of the phenomenon of positive biases when critiquing/utilizing research articles (Gray, 2001), are publication gap-reducing suggestions.

Hunting Gap

The hunting gap refers to difficulties in finding published research due to the limitations of current electronic databases (Gray, 2001). These limitations include limited database coverage and inadequate indexing of articles. Use of the Cochrane Library and improved search strategies can minimize the impact of this gap (Gray).

Quality Gap

The quality gap addresses the need for critical appraisal of evidence (Gray, 2001). Abstracts can be misleading in that they tend to be written with a bias toward highlighting the positive findings within a paper. In the search for evidence, it is essential to critique abstracts carefully—looking for structure, and carefully appraising the methods section—before accepting the results as good quality evidence. It is also important to be aware of sources of bias within research, and to critique the study design and presentation of results carefully (Gray).

The integrity and quality of an EBP as a policy fundamental is critical because an adopted policy has broad and far-reaching impact on health care delivery. Thus, to suggest or promote an EBP that has serious quality flaws as clinical evidence can lead to *serious* consequences for the researcher, organization, or policy-maker as well as for health delivery in general.

Evidence-based health policy may be viewed as the interface between evidence-based health care and public policy analysis (Lin, 2003). An evidence-based policy process should be guided by the collection of valid and reliable data, and following a process of determining the problem, developing a plan to address the problem, judging the feasibility of the plan, guiding the implementation of the plan, and then providing evidence from evaluation on which to base any needed future revisions (DePalma, 2002). However, policy too often is shaped by the interplay of political and philosophical differences. One must also recognize that policy-making is rarely a perfectly linear or systematic process. On the other hand, focusing on evidence in policy-making may allow those involved in the process a way to agree on a solution that is acceptable to all (DePalma). Attending to the policy problem by exploring the evidence of both the problem and its optional solutions may serve to reframe the debate away from entrenched philosophies toward application of scientific findings to finding new ways forward, thus nurturing sound, reasoned solutions.

CONCEPTUAL MODEL OF POLICY PROCESS: THE KINGDON MODEL

Researchers have developed models of agenda setting and policy formulation (Baumgartner & Jones, 1993; Cobb & Elder, 1983; Kingdon, 1995), while political scientists have developed theoretical modeling of policy design (Hedge & Mok, 1987). Ingraham noted the lack of one design, theory, or model in policy design (1987). Because of its applicability to health care, we have chosen the Kingdon Model for discussion in this work. Kingdon's Model is designed to answer two public policy questions: (1) how do issues get on the political agenda; and (2) once they are there, how are alternative solutions derived (Milstead, 1999). Kingdon's Model looks at both participants and processes involved in policy-making.

Policy participants can be interested parties either inside or outside of government and may include elected officials and their staff, political parties, special interest groups, professional organizations, or corporations, all of whom are disparate players. At a federal level, Kingdon ranks members of Congress second only to the President (the administration) in importance in agenda setting. He notes that members of Congress get involved to develop policy to meet their constituents' needs, to enhance their own political reputations with regard to ability and power, and to develop good policy to solve problems in which they are interested. According to Kingdon's model, elected officials are more important to agenda setting, whereas their staff members are more important to generating alternative solutions to policy problems. Kingdon asserts that special interest groups are more likely to block rather than promote a policy agenda item.

Kingdon's processes are conceived as three streams: problem streams, policy streams, and political streams. The problem stream includes ideas that get on an agenda if there are indicators of a problem or if there is inequity in the distribution of resources between groups of constituents. In the policy stream, officials push certain initiatives because of electoral reasons (from their party or their district) as well as belief in the worth of the initiative. In the policy stream, there are five criteria necessary for survival: (1) technical feasibility; (2) value acceptability within the policy community; (3) a cost that is acceptable or at least tolerable; (4) anticipated agreement from constituents; and (5) a reasonable chance that other elected decision-makers will be receptive to the initiative (Kingdon, 1995). The third stream (political) consists of elements such as upcoming elections, partisan distribution, ideological concerns in the policy-making body, and popular "mood" related to the problem or specific initiative.

In order for agenda setting to occur, there must be a coupling of streams during a critical time when a window of opportunity appears. According to Kingdon, "Policy windows open infrequently, and do not stay open long" (p. 166). Windows of opportunity can open either because there are new problems that have been brought to elected officials' attention or because of changes in the political stream, such as a newly elected administration or partisan power shifts after an election. Kingdon believes that the source of an idea is not as important as how it is nurtured: "Thus the key to understanding policy change is not where the idea came from but what made it take hold and grow" (p. 76). Kingdon's model is dynamic; "A problem is recognized, a solution is available, the political climate makes the time right for change, and the constraints do not prohibit action" (Kingdon, 1995, p. 93).

THE POLITICS OF EVIDENCE-BASED HEALTH POLICY

Policy-making at the state and federal levels is first and foremost a political process. Politics may be defined as "the process of influencing the allocation of scare resources" (Mason, Leavitt, & Chaffee, 2002, p. 9). Relatively few policy-makers at the state and federal levels have professional experience in the health care arena. For these policy-makers, their views are framed from personal experiences with the health care system or from anecdotal stories from their constituents. Policy-makers must balance competing agendas, claims, and spheres of influence when making policy decisions. Decisions may be influenced by politicians, party politics, campaign strategies, lobbyists, consumer groups, industries, media, and public opinion.

Evidence about the merits of a solution is but one aspect to be considered in the policy process. Policy-makers must also integrate values, cost, resources, and benefits (Gray, 2001; Sturm, 2002) at a population level. Gray acknowledges that "the clinician has to take into account the condition and values of the individual patient; that the policymaker has to take into account not only best current knowledge but also the needs of the populations, the values, the resources available, and the opportunity costs of the decision" (p. 371). Policy decisions are difficult, and the dynamics are more layered and complex than those in clinical care. Difficulty in reaching resolution on the "right" policy often results from a conflict between differing realms of influence such as ethical, social, cultural, economic, and electoral concerns and considerations (Black, 2001). Even with strength of evidence, policies may be made that run contrary to the evidence base.

Two such oppositional health policy examples come to mind. In 1988, the Office of Technology Assessment released a report documenting strong fiscal and clinical evidence that, in less than a year, a $1.00 investment in prenatal care including maternal nutrition returned $3.38 spent on care of low birth weight babies in neonatal intensive care. The 100th Congress appeared oblivious to these numbers and limited federal funding for pregnant women in the Women, Infants and Children supplemental nutrition program. That same Congress, again presented with even more data (evidence) on the value of good nutrition for growth and development in children, voted to count catsup as a green or yellow vegetable in the public school food supplement programs. What do these examples say? Surely their message is that much more is valued in policy than facts, data, evidence, or even just "because it is the right thing to do." Ideology, economics, debate over the size and role of government, winners, and losers are just a few of the factors that may impact policy decisions and products.

Obstacles Faced by Policy-Makers

Just like clinicians, policy-makers are presented with a number of challenges when trying to formulate health policy using EBP, including the multiple definitions of evidence, the difficulty of searching for evidence, the complexities of evaluating or grading the evidence, coupled with the nuances of the policy process. Policy-makers and their overworked staffs are challenged to understand the nuances in the criteria and to equate or compare levels of evidence from one schema to another. Therefore, it is incumbent upon those, such as health professionals, wishing to influence the policy decision-making process to conduct the search for evidence, present the evidence in an easy-to-understand format and completely honest and transparent manner, and look for ways to have evidence become high priority on the political agenda.

Lin suggests that policy results as a response to a perceived need or problem that is contingent upon the context in which the perceived need or problem occurs. Thus, EBP is made relevant in policy when the problem and its solutions—quality of care, technology dispersion, cost of care, and so on—provide the context.

Questions that are generated as a result of the policy-making process are inherently different than those questions that may be asked and answered as part of a clinical randomized controlled trial (RCT). Large numbers of persons are directly or indirectly affected by policy decisions at the state and federal levels. The general population represents a heterogeneous group and does not fit into a trial model of efficacy even under ideal circumstances.

Policy-makers are not likely to be experts at evaluating evidence per se. Haynes (1999) promotes three questions to be utilized to evaluate health care interventions (based on the work of A. Cochrane, a British epidemiologist): (1) "Can it work? (2) Does it work? (3) Is it worth it?" The question "can it work" addresses efficacy, or the extent to which the intervention does more good than harm under ideal circumstances. "Does it work" answers the question of effectiveness, or the extent to which the intervention works under usual or common circumstances. Answering the question "is it worth it" measures the outcomes of the intervention compared to the resources consumed (Haynes). The policy picture becomes cloudy when the answer to "can it work" conflicts with the findings of "is it worth it." At this point of balancing, the policy-maker is most susceptible to the other spheres of policy-shaping influences, including economics, politics, philosophies, and values.

Atkins, Siegel, and Slutsky (2005) have offered a framework for evaluation by policy-makers when the evidence is in dispute in order to assist in separating questions and concerns over the evidence from the other spheres or influence. Their framework consists of the following questions:

- What is the ultimate goal, and how does the intervention achieve those ends?
- How good is the evidence that the intervention can improve outcomes?
- How good is the evidence that the intervention will work in my setting?
- How do the potential benefits compare with the possible harms or costs of the intervention?

- What constitutes "good enough" evidence for a policy decision?
- What other considerations are relevant to policy decisions?

INTENDED AND UNINTENDED CONSEQUENCES

Policy-makers work toward policy with intended outcomes. The intended outcomes of EBP in health policy development are meritorious and much needed. EBP should be able to tell good science from bad; improve quality of care; decrease the costs of care; make technology diffusion both rational and rapid; and embrace multidisciplinary and systematic approaches to solving complex care problems. Together, these are both the promises of EBPs and their intended outcomes.

However, many unintended consequences occur in health policy. We have come to recognize that EBP may raise further examples of the unintended consequences of policy decisions. Thus, unintended results can negate positive outcomes of the evidence-based policy, complicating far-ranging treatment preferences among medical professionals and payment issues within insurance coverage. Several factors may contribute to this phenomenon, including inconsistent evidence from RCTs, lack of evidence from RCTs and cost considerations. Despite best intentions to predict and control the effect of any policy, it is difficult for decision-makers to foresee all consequences. These unintended consequences can have dramatic effects on the availability of services and procedures throughout the system.

A notable example of policy and the law of unintended consequences is the implementation of the Health Insurance Portability and Accountability Act of 1996 (HIPAA). Portability of insurance as one moves from job to job, privacy of medical information, and accountability of the health care system were all well-intentioned goals of the policy-makers who enacted HIPAA. However, unintended consequences abound with the implementation of the Administrative Simplification Compliance Act of 2001 (ASCA). ASCA has provisions for administrative simplification rules aimed at streamlining administrative processes of care through the implementation of transaction standards, privacy standards, and security standards. However, the reality is that these simplification rules are anything but simple.

As an example, the privacy regulations require all health care entities—including providers, health plans, and health data clearinghouses—to protect all patient information and to release minimum necessary information only after obtaining the appropriate patient consent. The regulation extended far beyond electronic medical information (as originally intended) to include oral and written communication and records as well. There is disagreement about the resulting balance between the rights of patients to privacy and the rights of the health professionals who use the information to improve care of the patients (Langner, 2001). Health care providers and entities have been faced with innumerable challenges of HIPAA implementation, such as increasing costs of health care business processes; increased documentation requirements around release of information; increased staffing needs such as hiring of institutional privacy officers; training and education of all levels of staff; and health service delivery delays due to difficulties that arise as clinical information is shared between providers when conflicting understandings of "minimum necessary" arise. Challenges also exist when communications with families must occur. These are but a few examples where the balance between patient rights and the challenges of complying with the regulations conflict. Few—if any—providers, health facilities, health plans, or business associates have been free from the unintended consequences of HIPAA.

In theory, all health care policies would be derived from the settled results of unflawed clinical trials. These trials should tell us whether a particular drug, procedure, or service is effective among the target audience and is superior or inferior to all other treatment choices. However, the reality is far more complicated. Similar clinical trials can have vastly different results. The trials might show benefits among select participants, but be unable to identify future users who might benefit from the service. Such was the case for implantable cardioverter defibrillators (ICD), where studies could not conclusively classify which persons at risk would benefit from an ICD (Hlatky, Sanders, & Owens, 2005). Because of these inconsistencies, the industry disagreed on the effectiveness of the procedure, although it did help a significant number of persons in the trial. As a result, insurance coverage on this procedure was restricted to persons with a certain kind of medical history (Hlatky et al.). This EBP example illustrates how the differences among trials can change reimbursement and insurance coverage for procedures and, therefore, the accessibility of those procedures to the public.

The reliance on evidence-based policies can negatively affect important interventions that lack sufficient trials and data to prove their effectiveness and value. RCTs can take several years to complete in order to have enough data to satisfy standards of grading. Emerging technologies and practices in many fields are moving at a much faster pace, and it is impossible for researchers to keep up with the development of these new services. Thus, if reimbursement or insurance coverage is based only on the accepted EBP, many new treatments could be stalled for several years until there is sufficient evidence, and promising practices may never be fleshed out. Furthermore, there are not enough EBPs to cover all available treatments in every specialty of care.

For example, mental health care is utilizing only six nationally recognized EBPs. The scope of these six practices in no way meets the needs of the field, the illnesses, or the many valid treatment possibilities. Therefore, any policy-making that would limit reimbursement to *only* those services based on EBPs could have serious consequences on persons who could benefit from the services considered "promising" or "best," but have not been fully vetted as evidence-based.

Finally, EBPs are not determined solely on their effectiveness and available data. Financial considerations can deter or promote certain health care policies over others. To return to the ICD example, insurance coverage was restricted not only because of the inconsistent trial results, but also due to the large cost of the procedure in conjunction with the significant number of persons at risk (Hlatky et al., 2005). The potential cost of covering this procedure is enormous.

Drug formularies can also be affected by policy decisions based on finances. Although the intent of a drug formulary is to lower the cost of drug therapies, it could be difficult if not impossible to add newer and often more expensive drugs to the formulary, even when the more expensive drug is a more effective treatment. EBPs could be an enormous plus in some situations (i.e., an expensive drug regime compared to re-hospitalization costs), yet getting there is long, arduous, and filled with both the EBP issues as well as the vagaries of health policy development. As a consequence, consumers may receive lower quality care waiting for either EBP or promising "breakthrough" practices to develop/inform health policy.

CONCLUSION

The use of EBPs in health policy has a long way to go. Just because EBP may be "the way of the now and the future" in the delivery of clinical health care, it is not certain that EBP is "the way" in health policy development. Actually, considering the complexities and uncertainties of the state of the "science" of EBP as described throughout this text, it is likely that many policy-makers will remain on the sidelines in calling for EBP to inform health policy.

REFERENCES

Atkins, D., Siegel, J., & Slutsky, J. (2005). Making policy when the evidence is in dispute. *Health Affairs, 24*(1), 102–113.

Baumgartner, F. R., & Jones, B. D. (1993). *Agendas and Instability in American Politics.* Chicago, IL: University of Chicago Press.

Black, N. (2001). Evidence-based policy: Proceed with care. *British Medical Journal, 323*(7307), 275–279.

Cobb, R. W., & Elder, C. D. (1983). *Participation in America: The Dynamics of Agenda-Building,* 2nd ed. Baltimore, MD: Johns Hopkins University Press.

DePalma, J. A. (2002). Proposing an evidence-based policy process. *Nursing Administration Quarterly, 26*(4), 55–61.

DePalma, J. A. (2004). Health policy and research: Evidence-based decision making. *Home Health Care Management and Practice, 16,* 405–407.

Eulau, H., & Prewitt, K. (1973). *Labyrinths of Democracy.* Indianapolis, IN: Bobbs-Merrill.

Evidence-Based Medicine Working Group (EBMWG). (1992). Evidence-based medicine: A new approach to teaching the practice of medicine. *Journal of the American Medical Association, 268*(17), 2420–2425.

Gerrish, K., & Clayton, J. (1998). Improving clinical effectiveness through an evidence-based approach: Meeting the challenge for nursing in the United Kingdom. *Nursing Administration Quarterly, 22*(4), 55–65.

Goode, C. J., & Piedalue, F. (1999). Evidence-based clinical practice. *Journal of Nursing Administration, 29*(6), 15–21.

Gray, J. A. Muir. (2001). *Evidence-Based Health Care: How to Make Health Policy and Management Decisions,* 2nd ed. London, UK: Churchill Livingstone.

Haynes, B. (1999). Can it work? Does it work? Is it worth it? *British Medical Journal, 319*(7211), 652–653.

Hedge, D. M., & Mok, J. W. (1987). The nature of policy studies: A content analysis of policy journal articles. *Policy Studies Journal, 16,* 49–62.

Htlaky, M. A., Sanders, G. D., & Owens, D. K. (2005). Evidence-based medicine and policy: The case of the implantable cardioverter defibrillator. *Health Affairs, 24*(1), 42–51.

Ingersoll, G. L. (2000). Op Ed. Evidence-based nursing: What it is and what it isn't. *Nursing Outlook, 48*(4), 151–152.

Ingraham, P. W. (1987). Toward more systematic consideration of policy design. *Policy Studies Journal, 15,* 611–628.

Jennings, B. M., & Loan, L. A. (2001). Misconceptions among nurses about evidence-based practice. *Journal of Nursing Scholarship, 33*(2), 121–127.

Jones, C. O. (1984). *An Introduction to the Study of Public Policy,* 2nd ed. Monterey, CA: Brooks-Cole.

Kingdon, J. W. (1995). *Agendas, Alternatives and Public Policies.* New York, NY: Harper Collins.

Langner, B. (2001). Unintended consequences: An inherent risk in public policy development. *Journal of Professional Nursing, 17*(2), 69–70.

Lasswell, H. D. (1958). *Politics: Who Gets What, When, How.* New York, NY: Meridian Books.

Lin, V. (2003). Competing rationalities: Evidence-based health policy? In V. Lin & B. Gibson (Eds.), *Evidence-Based Health Policy: Problems and Possibilities,* pp. 3–17. South Melbourne, Victoria, Australia: Oxford University Press.

Lohr, K. N., & Carey, T. S. (1999). Assessing the 'best evidence': Issues in grading the quality of studies for systematic reviews. *Joint Commission Journal of Quality Improvement, 25*(9), 470–479.

Mason, D., Leavitt, J. K., & Chaffee, M. W. (2002). Policy and politics, a framework for action. In D. Mason, J. K. Leavitt, & M. W. Chaffee (Eds.), *Policy and Politics in Nursing and Health Care,* pp. 1–18. St. Louis, MO: W. B. Saunders.

Milio, N. (1989). Developing nursing leadership in health policy. *Journal of Professional Nursing*, *5*(6), 315–321.

Milstead, J. A. (Ed). (1999). Advanced practice nurses and public policy, naturally. In *Health Policy and Politics*, pp. 1–41. Gaithersburg, MD: Aspen Publishers.

Rosenberg, W., & Donald, A. (1995). Evidence-based medicine: An approach to clinical problem-solving. *British Medical Journal*, *310*(6987), 1122–1126.

Sackett, D. L., Rosenberg, W. M. C., Gray, J. A. M., Haynes, R. B., & Richardson, W. S. (1996). Evidence-based medicine: What it is and what it isn't (Editorial). *British Medical Journal*, *312*(7023), 71–72.

Steinberg, E. P., & Luce, B. R. (2005). Evidence-based? Caveat emptor! *Health Affairs*, *24*(1), 80–92.

Stevens, K. R., & Paugh, J.A. (1999). Evidence-based practice and perioperative nursing. *Seminars in Perioperative Nursing*, *8*(3), 155–159.

Sturm, R. (2002). Evidence-based health policy versus evidence-based medicine. *Psychiatric Services*, *53*(12), 1499.

Sudduth, A. L. (1999). Policy evaluation. In J. A. Milstead (Ed.), *Health Policy and Politics*, pp. 219–256. Gaithersburg, MD: Aspen Publishers.

West, S., King, V., Carey, T. S., Lohr, K. N., McKoy N., Sutton, S. F., & Lux, L. (2002). *Systems to Rate the Strength of Scientific Evidence. Evidence Report/Technology Assessment No. 47.* (Prepared by the Research Triangle Institute-University of North Carolina Evidence-Based Practice Center under Contract No. 290-97-0011.) AHRQ Publication No. 02-E016. Rockville, MD: Agency for Healthcare Research and Quality. Available at http://www.ahrq.gov/clinic/tp/strengthtp.htm. Accessed March 2005.

CHAPTER 10

Creating Nursing System Excellence Through the Forces of Magnetism

Amy Steinbinder and Elaine Scherer

Just as clinical decision-making based on evidence is necessary for effective patient care, organizational decision-making based on evidence is vital for effective nursing services operations. This chapter presents expertise, best practices, and research findings related to evidence-based workplaces. Research findings identifying workplace attributes that were strongly linked to recruiting and retaining the best and brightest nurses were first published by the American Academy of Nursing in 1983 (McClure, Poulin, Sovie, & Wandelt), which was the original "magnet hospital study." The attributes, or "Forces of Magnetism" (FOM; Table 10.1) as they have come to be known, differentiated high performing organizations from others. These FOM and their relationship to evidence-based practice and achieving nursing system excellence are explored in this chapter.

In 1991, the American Nurses Credentialing Center (ANCC) introduced the Magnet Hospital Recognition Program for Excellence in Nursing Services, which included the initial FOM. The American Nurses Association's (ANA) *Standards for Organized Nursing Services* was used as the framework of the program (ANA, 1991). Many program changes have occurred since 1991 that are based on research, evidence-based practices, and consensus opinions of experts and other recognized authorities, including the International Organization for Standardization. Since its inception, the Magnet Recognition Program has awarded Magnet designation to over 140 organizations; the latest listing can be found on the Magnet program Web site (www.nursecredentialing.org) (ANCC, 2003).

The Magnet Recognition Program has been highly visible over the past 10 years. Not only is magnet designation known to and desired by nursing leaders and nursing staffs, but it is becoming a highly prized goal of hospital chief executive officers (CEOs) and health care system leaders to attract physicians, develop market excellence, and recruit clinical staff. The public also is becoming aware

Table 10.1   Fourteen Forces of Magnetism

Force of Magnetism	Expectations of the Magnet Environment[1]
Quality of Nursing Leadership	Nurse leaders are knowledgeable, strong, visionary risk-takers. They advocate and support staff and patients. Their philosophy is clear, well-articulated, and guides day-to-day operations of the nursing services.
Organizational Structure	The structure is characterized as flat and decentralized. Shared decision-making is functioning and productive. The structure is dynamic and responsive to change. Nursing is present and actively involved in organizational committees. The chief nursing officer (CNO) reports to the CEO, and executive level nursing leaders serve at the executive level of the organization.
Management Style	A participative management style is pervasive and staff feedback is encouraged, valued, and used by leaders in decision-making. Nursing leaders are visible, accessible, and communicate effectively with staff.
Personnel Policies and Programs	Salaries and benefits are competitive. Staffing and scheduling systems are flexible and creative. Evidence-based staffing based on acuity is expected. Staff nurses are involved in creating personnel policies and programs that support professional nursing practice, work/life balance, and delivery of quality care.
Professional Models of Care	Care models give nurses responsibility and authority to provide patient care. In addition, nurses are accountable for coordinating care and ensuring that continuity of care is provided across the continuum. Patients' unique needs are addressed to achieve desired outcomes.
Quality of Care	Staff nurses perceive that care provided is high-quality. Positive patient outcomes are achieved. Patient safety, ethical practice, research, and evidence-based practice are included.
Quality Improvement	Structures and processes are in place to measure quality and improve care and service to patients. Staff nurses actively participate in improvement activities and gain knowledge in the process.

Table 10.1   Fourteen Forces of Magnetism (*continued*)

Force of Magnetism	Expectations of the Magnet Environment[1]
Consultation and Resources	Experts including advance practice nurses are available to staff. Nurses are encouraged to participate in professional organizations.
Autonomy	Nurses are expected to use independent judgment in providing appropriate care for patients. An interdisciplinary approach to care is expected and nursing care is consistent with professional standards and scope of practice.
Community and the Health Care Organization	A strong community presence is maintained, and outreach programs are offered that benefit the community.
Nurses as Teachers	Nurses include teaching in their practice that includes patient education and precepting/mentoring new graduates and students as well as experienced nurse colleagues.
Image of Nursing	Nursing services are perceived as essential by other members of the health care team. Nurses are integral to care and are recognized as vital contributors to care delivery.
Interdisciplinary Relationships	Collaborative relationships and mutual respect are evident throughout the organization as all members of the health care team contribute to achieving clinical outcomes.
Professional Development	Education is a high priority and includes orientation, in-service programs, continuing education, formal education, and career development. Clinical and leadership competencies are valued, and nurses have opportunity to obtain national specialty certifications as well as participate in clinical career advancement programs.

[1]As defined by the Expert Panel for *2005 Magnet Application Manual.*

of Magnet designation. The Governor of Vermont, Howard Dean, M.D., recognized Southwestern Vermont Medical Center's Magnet achievement when it was the 47th Nursing Service to achieve the designation (www.svhealthcare.org). *The Readers Digest* recommended that patients "would be foolish" not to check into a Magnet hospital if one was located nearby (Pekkanen, 2003, p. 91).

The 14 FOM have been well researched over the last 20 years and continue to be subject to major scrutiny. The ANCC Commission on Magnet recently completed a thorough evaluation of the application procedures and has restructured the process around the FOM (ANCC, 2004a). This comprehensive review brought in nursing experts from around the country, including nurse leaders, academicians, advanced practice nurses, staff nurses, nurse managers, experienced magnet appraisers, chief nurse executives (CNEs) and their representatives, researchers, psychomatricians, and previous leaders in the Magnet program. These leaders were brought to the ANCC offices and also gathered in multiple conference calls regarding the process. The manual was then released in draft format, giving the Commission the opportunity to hear public comment. This commitment to ensuring an evidence-based process is critical to maintaining the integrity of the program and is the primary goal of the Magnet Commission.

OVERVIEW

For this chapter, three sources of information were used to provide evidence demonstrating the relationship of magnet designation to system excellence. First, ten Chief Nurse Officers (CNOs) of magnet designated organizations who served as magnet program implementation experts were interviewed in depth by the co-authors (Table 10.2). These CNOs candidly discussed their hospitals' journey and provided specific examples of programs that led to magnet designation. Second, a literature search was performed, which interestingly supported many of the findings gleaned from the CNOs' interviews. Third, best practices cited in the *Best Practices in Today's Challenging Health Care Environment* (ANCC, 2004b) were the final source of information used to link magnet designation to system excellence.

The 14 FOM identified in the original magnet study were discussed, as were their relationships to the "Eight Essentials of Magnetism" identified by Kramer as the elements of giving high quality patient care that were most important to staff nurses (Kramer & Schmalenberg, 2002). Interviewer stories and insights were highlighted with each FOM.

The demographic characteristics of the interviewed CNOs and their organizations are described. Each FOM is discussed, and pertinent literature supporting

Table 10.2 Chief Nursing Officer, Hospital Affiliation, and Original Designation Date of Facility

CNO, Credentials and Title	Hospital Affiliation and Location	Original Magnet Designation Date
Rebecca Burke, RN, MS Vice President for Patient Care Services/Chief Nursing Officer	The Miriam Hospital Providence, Rhode Island	January 1998
Linda Deering, MSN, RN Vice President & Chief Nursing Officer	Delnor Community Hospital Geneva, Illinois	February 2004
Toni Fiori, MA, RN, CNAA Executive Vice President/ Patient Care and Chief Nursing Officer	Hackensack University Medical Center, Hackensack, New Jersey	February 1995
Marie Golanowski, RN, MS, CNAA Regional Vice President/ Chief Nurse Executive	Aurora Health Care, Metro Region, - St. Luke's Medical Center, St. Luke's South Shore Hospital, Aurora Sinai Medical Center, West Allis Memorial Hospital and Aurora Medical Center-Washington County, Wisconsin	January 2001
Val Gokenback, RN, MBA, CNA Administrative Director, Chief Nurse Executive	William Beaumont Hospital Royal Oak, Michigan	January 2004
Susan Grant, MS, RN, CNAA, BC Chief Nursing Officer and Associate Administrator for Patient Care Services	University of Washington Seattle, Washington	May 1994
Craig Luzinski, MS, RN Vice President of Patient Care Services/Chief Nurse Executive	Poudre Valley Health System Fort Collins, Colorado	June 2000

Table 10.2   Chief Nursing Officer, Hospital Affiliation, and Original Designation Date of Facility (*continued*)

CNO, Credentials and Title	Hospital Affiliation and Location	Original Magnet Designation Date
Debra Mals, RN, MS Vice President Hospital Operations, Chief Nursing Officer	Miami Valley Hospital Dayton, Ohio	June 2004
Vickie Moore, MSN, RN, CHE, CNAA, BC Senior Vice President, Operations	St. Joseph's Hospital Atlanta, Georgia	May 2000
Mary Wicker, MS, RN Vice President of Operations	Southwestern Vermont Medical Center Bennington, Vermont	March 2002

the force and its relationship to outcomes of organizational performance is included. Third, any evidence linking the FOM to one or more Essentials of Magnetism is identified. Finally, comments provided by the interviewed CNOs were included to illustrate the relationship of actual practice to research findings.

CHIEF NURSING OFFICER INTERVIEWS

The interviewed CNOs described their journeys toward achieving and then sustaining the prestigious magnet designation. CNOs were chosen based on type of facility, length of time it had been designated as a magnet organization, and geographic location of the hospital. Four of the CNOs were from large urban, academic-affiliated hospitals (Table 10.3). One individual was the CNO of a five-hospital system. One of the hospitals was a large tertiary care teaching facility in an urban setting. The remaining four facilities were community-based. Four of the CNOs were in community hospitals and one CNO was in a rural hospital. Four organizations are located in the Midwest, 3 in the East, 2 in the West, and 1 is in the South (Table 10.4). Six organizations achieved magnet status within three months to four years, and the remaining four sustained magnet designation for six to ten years. Three hospitals underwent two redesignations since their original designation, and one underwent a first redesignation (Table 10.5).

Table 10.3   Type of Hospital

	Tertiary/ Academic	5-Hospital System	Community	Rural
Number of hospitals	4	1	3	1

Table 10.4   Hospital Location

	East	Midwest	South	West
Number of hospitals	3	4	1	2

Table 10.5   Number of Years Designated as a Magnet Facility

	< 1 year	2–4 years	6–7 years	10 years
Number of hospitals	3	3	3	1

Six of the ten individuals were in their CNO role at the time of original designation (Table 10.6). Three CNOs who were not in the CNO role at the time of original designation were working in the organization at the time of designation. Only three of the individuals were hired external to the organization. Seven of the 10 CNOs were promoted into their CNO roles. In fact, these 10 individuals had 4.5 to 37 years of tenure in their organizations and were in the CNO role from 1 to 18 years. According to Collins (2001), who interviewed CEOs of companies generally regarded for their excellence to identify their differentiating attributes, 10 out of 11 good to great CEOs came from inside the company. This finding is similar to the CNO interviewees, where the majority of CNOs were promoted from within their organizations.

Only two of the organizations had undergone a merger. Three had a change in CEO. Four CNOs described their roles as expanding over the years from operational accountability for nursing only to accountability for many or all clinical departments. One organization transitioned from being a community-based to a tertiary care-based provider, and one organization underwent a significant change in both strategic direction and key leadership due to financial instability that occurred after initial designation. This organization did sustain magnet

Table 10.6   CNO Tenure at Current Magnet Facility

	Years as CNO			Years in Organization		
	1.5–5	6–7	12–18	2–5	6–15	19–37
Number of CNOs	6	2	2	3	4	3

status at the time of redesignation despite the reorganization that preceded redesignation.

A convenience sample was used and the interviews were limited to 30 to 45 minutes per CNO. Questions were provided in advance of the scheduled telephone interview, so that the nurse leaders could think about them ahead of time. Interviews were conducted over the summer months. Each CNO who was asked to participate agreed without hesitation and found time for the interview despite demanding schedules and a short scheduling time frame. Information gleaned from these articulate, knowledgeable leaders is shared throughout the discussion of the FOM.

FORCES OF MAGNETISM: EVIDENCE IN PRACTICE

Based on the literature, CNO interviews, and comparing the FOM with Kramer's Essentials of Magnetism, the following five FOM factors were found to be the most significantly linked to system excellence: quality of nursing leadership, quality of care, autonomy, professional development, and interdisciplinary relationships. Each is discussed, followed by the remaining nine FOMs.

Quality of Nursing Leadership

The quality of nursing leadership is the most significant FOM. Several studies illustrate the strong relationship of nursing leadership and the impact on work environment and organizational outcomes. In addition, nursing leadership influences each of Kramer's eight Essentials of Magnetism as evidenced by overlapping descriptors between quality of nursing leadership and each essential.

The 10 CNOs who were interviewed all identified nursing leadership as the number one FOM necessary to achieve magnet designation. Role modeling excellence, mentoring, coaching, maintaining high visibility, and inviting staff to

Table 10.7   Essentials of Magnetism

Working with other nurses who are clinically competent	Nurses stated in the study that "recognition and reward for clinical competence" was important, not the clinical ladder programs (p. 30). Clinical competence was one of four value themes identified by CNEs. Also, this is the factor most significantly correlated with perception of adequate staffing, job satisfaction, and perceived ability to give quality care.
Good RN–MD relationships and communication	These relationships are essential to magnetism. These relationships are essential to provide quality care and to nurse–physician collaborative practice programs. A five category scale identified to describe nurse–physician relationships beginning with the best includes collegial, collaborative, student-teacher, neutral and negative (p. 33).
Nurse autonomy and accountability	General definition of the concept of autonomy used in the study was the freedom to act on what you know (p. 36). Two additional dimensions were added: scope ("does practice relate to nursing care only or extend more broadly to patient care?") and sanction ("Is practice organizationally sanctioned?") (p. 36).
Supportive nurse manager, supervisor	The quality and support of the leadership team has been recognized as a central factor in the success of magnet hospitals, impacting job satisfaction, quality care, and attracting nurses to their facilities (p. 41). It is also essential for establishing and maintaining both nurse–physician collaborative practice and shared governance or some kind of control over nursing practice structure.
Control over nursing practice and practice environment	Identified by staff nurses as essential to giving quality care. Control over practice distinguished Magnets in prior research. Domains of control usually include clinical practice, management, quality control of practitioners, and education. One outcome of control over practice cited by many nurses was "increased status, respect, and recognition" (p. 43).

Table 10.7   Essentials of Magnetism (*continued*)

Support for education (in-service, continuing education)	The focus of support for education has changed from on-site BSN programs once attached to job satisfaction and effectiveness. Over the years it has become more varied, including tuition for short-term courses, internships, externships, and on-site BSN/MSN programs and in-service education that affects attraction and retention as well as job satisfaction and giving quality care (p. 43).
Adequate nurse staffing	In an organization where nurses perceive their coworkers as competent, "staff are able to work with less staff and oftentimes produce more and better quality nursing care because they are confident in one another's abilities and trust the work of their colleagues"(p. 30). Six indicators are routinely used to measure nurse shortage: vacancy rate, RN-to-patient ratio, turnover rate, use of supplemental staff, multiple applicants for available positions, and staff nurse perception of adequacy (p. 45).
Concern for the patient is paramount in this organization	A mark of excellence in organizations is the extent to which a system of common and shared core values is in place with values that go beyond the technical requirements of a job....when staff nurses have autonomy and trust management to listen, be responsive to, and have respect for role and value difference, a dynamic institution exists (p. 51).

Source: Used with permission from American Nurses Publishing. Kramer & Schmalenberg. (2002). *Magnet Hospitals Revisited: Attraction and Retention of Professional Nurses.*

dialogue with the CNO were identified again and again. Although these CNOs did not label themselves as risk takers, they told stories illustrating their risk-taking behaviors. Risk taking is a critical attribute of effective nurse leaders. For example, two CNOs described implementing shared governance in organizations where the senior leadership was skeptical. In fact, one team was adamantly opposed, as shared governance appeared to be a form of collective bargaining. The CNOs were confident, calm, prepared, and listened to concerns of leaders; they responded to concerns in a manner that garnered the CEOs' support initially and leadership's support subsequently.

Additionally, the magnet nurse leaders described the impact of rounding on patient care units and asking staff about their patient care assignments and staffing needs. Rounding provides CNOs the opportunity to observe barriers to care as well as to inquire about systems and processes that support nursing practice. Conversations between nurses and the CNO demonstrated to staff the importance of patient care, the nursing care delivery model, and the multidisciplinary approach to care. Nurses can discuss patient care and outcomes achieved, and CNOs can recognize staff for specific accomplishments.

Upenieks (2003) interviewed four CNOs (2 from magnet hospitals and 2 from nonmagnet hospitals) and 12 nurse leaders to identify both the significant attributes of effective nurse leaders and the organizational factors that support professional nursing practice. Two significant findings were (1) ability to judge merit of the newest nursing trend without being swayed and (2) ability to use data to develop a compelling case to change staffing mix and/or hours of care to meet patient needs. Upenieks' study findings are consistent with CNO interviews. For example, one CNO created an Office for Magnet Program by selecting two innovative educators to bring the Magnet process alive at the facility. Since no additional full-time equivalents had been built into the budget, the CNO's vision of achieving magnet designation was realized in a unique manner. She provided the educators with secretarial support, included them in initial planning, and then gave them freedom to implement the process in their own way. These two leaders successfully managed the plan from the beginning through to the Magnet site visit, and the result was Magnet designation for their facility.

This same CNO was asked to have nurses assume responsibility for transporting patients from the inpatient setting to another facility for radiation oncology procedures. The CNO demonstrated her patient advocacy and nursing leadership abilities by agreeing to conduct an investigation, and to report back to the senior leadership team who had requested the transport. She quickly mobilized the staff involved to conduct a time study and collect data to evaluate the efficiency and safety of the transport plan. As a result of the study, the relocation of the Radiation Oncology move did not occur because patient safety was compromised and the registered nurse (RN) time spent in transport was excessive. Her ability to provide objective data that were collected by nurses and valued by the senior leaders is an excellent example of using expertise and patient preferences to drive decision-making.

Despite distractions, CNOs demonstrated a tremendous aptitude for maintaining focus as they pursued magnet designation and/or redesignation. The ability to sustain passion, commitment, and energy was evident as one CNO described her organization's significant financial faltering following the intial magnet designation. Poor financial performance then occurred, 75 staff lost their jobs, and the nursing education department was depleted. Rebuilding the organization and re-establishing its culture took time and perseverance, which resulted in the facility achieving redesignation a few years later.

Other examples of the CNOs' focus and determination included incorporating key organizational strategies into their nursing department to align their goals to achieve Magnet status. For example, patient satisfaction as the primary organizational initiative, zero agency use, and changes in benchmark indicators were seen as congruent with the pursuit of Magnet designation. Even changes in key leaders, such as CEO or Human Resources Vice President, or changes in reporting structures could not dissuade the CNOs from achieving Magnet goals.

Neuhauser (2002) interviewed seven CNOs and identified 15 strategies implemented by nurse leaders to build a "high-retention culture." These strategies included: inspiring top performers; building a culture that embraced flexibility and adaptation; promoting from within as a reward for academic achievement; building relationships on all levels; teaching mentoring and coaching skills to front line managers; rounding; and having zero tolerance for inappropriate physician behavior and poor performers. These Neuhauser strategies were discussed by the CNOs interviewed for this chapter.

Several CNOs discussed the importance of weekly rounding in all patient care areas. One, Linda Deering, described herself as being accountable for outcomes achieved in all nursing areas. She stated that rounds are not optional. "If patient satisfaction scores are not what they should be, that tells me I am not rounding on leaders. I am not praising, enough. If I am visible to pump up our leaders, they then are able to be present for their staff and pump them up." Deering went on to say, "My calendar is a reflection of what I am getting for results. If I don't change the stuff on my calendar, I will continue getting the same results. It takes courage to change your calendar, but it is essential for success."

A recent study of 820 nurses from 40 units in 20 urban U.S. hospitals showed that the lack of administrative support of nursing care was a significant factor in nurses' emotional exhaustion, which is a component of nurse burnout and patient dissatisfaction (Vahey, Aiken, Sloane, Clarke, & Vargas, 2004). The three instruments used in that study are well validated and include: Nursing Work Index-Revised, a measure of nurses' practice environment; the Maslach Burnout Inventory, a nurse outcome measure; and the La Monica Oberst Patient Satisfaction Scale. Deering's (2004) rounding strategy is an ideal way to gauge staff nurses' ability to provide safe, effective care with minimal perceived barriers to practice.

Kleinman (2004) discussed the positive relationship of nurse retention and effective leadership, defined as those using transformational leadership behaviors. These behaviors included sharing a compelling vision, instilling a sense of pride, motivating staff, and encouraging staff to offer their ideas. All were directly related to staff satisfaction and ultimately nurse retention. These principles were clearly articulated by the interviewed CNOs.

Level 5 leadership was defined by Collins (2001) as the ability of leaders to stay focused on organizational success rather than personal recognition. Leaders who demonstrated this style were not highly charismatic or high-profile, but instead were selfless, understated leaders with a tremendous capacity to maintain focus and face the brutal facts of the current situation. Level 5 leaders are strategic thinkers and strategy makers. They are continuously scanning the horizon for innovative approaches to address current challenges. Moore (2004) gave great examples of her current and future programs designed to bring her vision into the present. She is developing a Center for Nursing Excellence through a capital campaign targeted to raise $2 million. The intent of this Center is to prepare for the next 20 years. Its research focus is patient outcomes related to nursing care and the environment in which nurses practice, with two priorities of supporting autonomy in practice and advocating for patients. Moore's dynamic concepts netted over $200,000 even before the campaign's planned kickoff.

Golanowski (2004) described an innovative partnership that her organization has formed with a prominent researcher from a local university and an electronic medical record software company to develop a database of clinical information to measure the impact of nursing care on patient outcomes. This new knowledge could then be used to identify best practices so they may be implemented on a much larger scale, perhaps even nationally.

Each CNO also discussed the vital role of nurse managers as leaders. Leadership was needed to support staff in developing the shared decision-making process at the unit level. Managers made rounds on patients on a consistent basis and were highly visible on their units. Managers observed staff members in their roles, praising them for good performance and not tolerating poor performance. These CNOs echoed Buckingham and Coffman's (1999) research of over a million employees in various industries: employees don't leave organizations, they leave their immediate supervisors.

Several CNOs described the formal leadership development programs that they implemented for their managers and staff. Luzinski (2004) brings 250 leaders together on a quarterly basis for a full day of education, discussion, and planning. Staff nurses who are promoted into manager positions are given formal management training to help them to be successful in their new roles. Staff nurses who are elected to shared governance councils participate in a comprehensive class to prepare them for their new roles as council members.

Quality of Care

"All nurses come to work to do their best."   Toni Fiore (2004)

There is a perception that nurses give high quality care in Magnet hospitals. Patient and nurse satisfaction surveys, along with nurse sensitive indicators, provide three of the means of measuring quality of care at Magnet facilities. These data are gathered, benchmarked nationally, and goals are set to continually improve. Interim monitoring data are collected by the ANCC, which annually monitors the quality data provided by the designated facilities (ANCC, 2004a). Poudre Valley's Craig Luzinski states that his facility has been a successful Magnet facility primarily because of its culture; they sell a "quality culture" and Poudre Valley is working for a 99% rating in customer satisfaction. This is true also for the Miriam's Rebecca Burke (2004), who stated that the Miriam hospital "had no wimpy goals."

All of the CNOs interviewed referred to quality of care as important to the success of their organization. This is supported by strong relationships of the components of the forces and the eight essentials. Clinically competent colleagues, control over practice and environment, autonomy, nurse–physician relationships, and concern for the patient had the strongest correlations. Kramer and Schmalenberg found that competence was the basis for organizationally sanctioned autonomy, for collegial nurse–physician relationships, and for effective control over practice (2002, p. 31). Professional cultures are enhanced by education level and professional nurses being at the bedside. One study found that a 10% increase in the proportion of nurses holding a bachelor's degree was associated with a 5% decrease in both the likelihood of patients dying within 30 days of admission and the odds of failure to rescue (Aiken, Clarke, Cheung, Sloane, & Silber, 2003). Forty-two percent of the nurses at Miami Valley Hospital are Baccalaureate level RNs, which has helped create a culture of excellence (Mals, 2004). At Meridian Health Systems, obtaining national certification within two years of employment is a standard (Hader, 2004). Many hospitals have developed core groups of nurses to help guide the improvement of care. RNs at North East Medical Center assume responsibility for prescribing, delegating, and coordinating nursing care (ANCC, 2004b).

There is strong integration of research and evidence-based practice with human and material resources to support care delivery. An excellent example is from St. Joseph's Hospital in Atlanta, Georgia. Vicki Moore (2004) is developing the Center for Nursing Excellence, with a PhD nurse position and a doctoral fellow to conduct and publish organizational research.

The Florida Magnet hospitals partnered with the University of South Florida College of Nursing (2004) to sponsor the "1st Annual Florida Magnet Nursing Research Conference." The Conference highlighted at least 30 poster presentations of research accomplished by nurses on their staff. The excitement exhibited by the nurses as they described their research and the subsequent impact it had on patient care were noted by all that attended.

Autonomy

Porter-O'Grady (2003) believes that shared governance is a structural model through which nurses can express and manage their practice with a higher level of professional autonomy. He has consulted with many hospitals that have since earned Magnet recognition, and two of the interviewed CNOs said that his assistance was instrumental in guiding their particular facility to incorporate the principles of shared governance.

The definition of clinical autonomy that best captures the staff nurses' viewpoint is: "the freedom to act on what you know, to make independent clinical decisions that exceed standard nursing practice, in the best interest of the patient" (Kramer & Schmalenberg, 2002). The original research examined many creative and innovative programs that evolved when nurses were given the freedom and accountability to be autonomous (McClure & Hinshaw, 2002). While autonomy was not the primary force or essential factor identified as being most important in our interviews, it was mentioned multiple times as a key component, and CNOs definitely perceive it as their responsibility to support. It is important that nursing determines the practice of nursing both individually at the bedside and organizationally in support for staff (Golanowski, 2004). The relationship to other forces and essentials was evident with the understanding that it is essential to have nurses involved in research for autonomy (Fiore, 2004) as well as policies and programs to enhance autonomy (Gokenbeck, p. 31, 2004). Control over practice has a lot to do with shared governance and empowering nurses (Mals, 2004), and "the most important is autonomy" (Moore, 2004). A nurse-run clinic at Meridian Health Systems for congestive heart failure patients has been successful in improving the lives of patients by decreasing hospitalizations and clinic visits, thereby saving over 1 million dollars in three years (Hader, 2004).

Building magnetism into hospitals is the subject of a chapter written by Ada Sue Hinshaw in *Magnet Hospitals Revisited* (McClure & Hinshaw, 2002), which lists potential strategies to enhance autonomy. The most telling statement in the chapter is that, *"while the strategies are relatively straightforward, the necessary environment is more difficult to develop. The major issue is building trust in the clinical setting for nurses to take actions that may be risky and may both succeed or fail* (p. 94)." Autonomous practice is a highly evolved clinical attribute. Nurses need to be coached and mentored to demonstrate autonomy in their practice. CNOs can nurture autonomous practice by verbally and publicly recognizing nurses when they have taken the initiative to act on behalf of a patient. In the event that a nurse's autonomous act does not achieve the desired outcome, it is essential that the CNO or nurse manager support the nurse's action and discuss the situation together to assist the nurse in learning from the situation. The nurse's willingness to take autonomous action must be recognized in a positive manner even though the expected result was not achieved. This type of interaction builds trust and demonstrates that taking action on behalf of a patient is always supported regardless of the outcome.

Organizational Structure: Integrating Context

Reporting structures in organizations provides valuable information regarding the involvement of the CNO in key decision-making forums. CNOs, who report directly to CEOs, are voting members of the finance, strategic planning, and other executive level committees within the organization. They not only have a voice at the table but are able to influence the direction and resources of the hospital (ANCC, 2004a). CNOs attend Board meetings and report on status of nursing. Active involvement on Medical Executive Committees allows the CNO to develop collaborative, collegial relationships with medical staff leadership. A flat, decentralized organizational structure provides flexibility and supports innovation at the unit and department level.

Tonges, Baloga-Altieri, and Atzori (2004) described the Nurse Practice Committee (NPC), a self-management structure, as a mechanism to review practice, propose innovative approaches to support care delivery, and promote communication and collegial relationships among nurses. This structure empowered staff, as evidenced by implementation of programs resulting in significant outcomes. For example, scheduling practices were modified, resulting in retention of nurses who had expressed intent to leave the organization and creation of several new positions including a night transport technician, a telemetry transport team, an RN expeditor position to admit patients from the emergency department, nursing retention coordinator, and an evening/night shift education specialist. The CNO secured a substantial budget to support these innovations. In addition, proposed projects, once approved by the NPC, were not subject to any other additional approval processes. Nurses involved in improving their work environment, who experience autonomy and control over practice in the process, express a strong sense of ownership, which is the desired outcome of shared governance.

Operationalizing shared governance within the nursing department is feasible in an organization where the CNO has the authority to initiate demonstration projects. Shared governance is a structure and process that embodies the principles of equity, partnership, accountability, and ownership, which are necessary for autonomy to flourish (Porter-O'Grady, 2003). Organizations, while incorporating shared governance as the vehicle for nurses to manage their own practice, empower staff and create the culture where nurses want to practice.

The active involvement and support of the CEO was identified as a critical success factor to achieve and sustain success. One CNO stated that she partnered with her CEO to build a culture of empowerment. Although shared governance was not totally understood by the senior leadership team, the CEO supported the CNO in creating and implementing the model in the hospital. His belief was that if something was best for the patient, he would support it. Another CNO stated that her organization had been very stable and change was approached cautiously. The CEO demonstrated his belief in the strength of nursing leadership by supporting the CNO's proposal to implement the NPC and shared-decision making by nurses, even though other members of the senior leadership team did not want to pursue the new approach.

CNOs reinforced the need for flat, nonhierarchical organizational structures by indicating that flat structures allow for agility, interaction, and various approaches to achieving outcomes. CNOs described several activities they engage in to ensure their visibility and their first-hand knowledge of staff concerns. These include formal CNO rounds on all shifts and all units every month, focus groups of staff to gain in-depth understanding of specific issues (i.e., retention strategies, changes in staffing practices, and new program implementation); and open forums to facilitate information sharing and to obtain feedback. Communication among staff and their managers is improved. Involving staff in decision-making through shared governance is necessary as is budgeting for staff, so that their time on councils and committees is compensated.

Gokenback (2004) described a unique nursing organizational structure in which four CNEs have equal authority and power. One CNE is appointed chairperson by the CEO. This individual is the single voice of nursing and is the CNE who attends the Board meetings. All nursing and ancillary departments report to the CNEs. Golanowski (2004) stated that the chairperson of Aurora Health Care–Metro Region System Shared Governance Council is a voting member of the system-level CNO structure and participates in the strategic planning session.

Several of the CNOs hired a consultant to work with the nursing leadership team and ultimately the nursing staff to create a shared governance structure that would meet the needs of the organization. Each CNO identified the value of shared governance in building a professional, engaged work force that is responsive, responsible, and accountable for the practice of nursing. Although each of the 10 CNOs described a shared governance structure with unit-based councils, the actual councils/committees comprising shared governance were varied.

Management Style

Leaders who are attentive to being visible and accessible have the opportunity to engage in informal dialogue with staff. These leaders are able to observe system and process issues that are barriers to nursing practice. They are in a position to ask staff, "What required too many hand-offs today?" and "what kept you from doing your best work today?" Buckingham and Coffman (1999) described a management style in which managers motivate by focusing on individuals' strengths, coaching people to help them find the right fit within the organization, and setting clear expectations for staff, not the steps, but the outcomes so that staff will be engaged and successful in the organization. Staff members do not leave organizations; they leave their immediate supervisors, so managing in an open, collaborative manner while clearly delineating expectations, supports professional nursing practice.

Horton-Deutsch and Wellman (2002) revisited Christman's principles for effective management that were first published in 1982. These principles were revalidated for nurse managers today. Having the skill to establish a just reward system to retain competent caregivers, inspire innovative approaches to practice, apply appropriate theories to practice to enhance care, and quantify nursing care to demonstrate nursing's contribution to patient outcomes, continue to be important leadership principles that were also reinforced during the CNO interviews.

Knowing how to accept, foster, and delegate accountability to retain staff and build a just culture is another area requiring expertise on the part of nurse leaders (Horton-Deutsch & Wellman, 2002; Marx, 2001; Neuhauser, 2002). Identifying the key actions and outcomes for each leader, manager, and staff nurse is necessary to focus each individual on what is expected of them. Developing written performance agreements is one concrete way for the manager and employee to discuss expectations so there will be no surprises at the time of the individual's annual performance evaluation.

Shared governance is congruent with a participative management style. If nurse managers are consistent in their ability to clarify the work, delineate the outcomes, and establish clear boundaries, staff nurses will engage in partnering to resolve problems and conflict. Managers who communicate often, anticipate and address potential barriers, and who are willing to be hands-on to provide support and demonstrate shared values, actively cultivate a professional nursing practice environment.

The ability to directly measure staff nurses' perception of actual versus preferred involvement in decision-making may provide managers and leaders insight about the nursing practice environment (Havens & Vasey, 2003). Their Decisional Involvement Scale (DIS) was developed to identify involvement in six areas related to professional work environment: (1) unit staffing; (2) quality of professional practice; (3) recruitment; (4) unit governance and leadership; (5) quality of support staff practice; and (6) collaboration. Managers and leaders interested in providing nurses with opportunities to become actively involved in unit-based decisions could use the DIS as a baseline measure of involvement, and then as a measure of success following implementation of staff nurse involvement strategies.

All 10 CNOs described in their own words that the shared governance/ shared leadership/shared decision-making model is the cornerstone of the nursing department's culture. Staff nurses are not only encouraged, but they are expected to engage in unit-based council activities that impact nursing practice. Staff nurses are actively involved in making decisions about their practice. Implementing shared governance occurs over time. Based on expert opinion, a minimum of two years is required to initiate the model, and the journey often takes several more years before it is operating smoothly, effectively, and efficiently.

Staff nurses need leadership education to understand their roles in this model (Golanowski, 2004). Staff nurses who begin serving on practice councils and other shared governance councils do not know how to represent nursing in general. They come to meetings prepared only to give their own perspectives. Through education and coaching, they become well versed in ways of effectively obtaining needed input and feedback from colleagues prior to meetings, so that the decision-making process is not bogged down. Several CNOs brought in experts to assist the organization in creating and implementing their shared governance models.

Personnel Policies and Procedures

Staffing

Adequate nurse staffing is an essential component of magnetism that attracts and retains nurses at the bedside (Upenieks, 2003; Kramer & Schmalenberg, 2002). Evidence of this component is included in several of the FOM, but it is most directly addressed in the Personnel Policies and Procedures force, which identifies the staffing and scheduling system as adapting and flexing to factors in the environment to support safe patient care. Staffing concerns accounted for 76% of nurses' leaving one health care system in Iowa (Strachota, Normandin, O'Brien, Clary, & Krukow, 2003).

Scheduling

Flexible schedules are another retention strategy (Upenieks, 2003). Nurses want versatility and respond by continuing their employment in the organization that meets this need. Access to employee assistance programs and Human Resources personnel in the event of concerns and complaints is also available. Gokenbach (2004) stated that her organization has adapted a zero tolerance abuse policy. This policy is supported by all leadership and protects staff from any potential negative interpersonal conflicts.

Patient Classification

Dynamic staffing systems that are based on patient acuity are ideal, as recommended staffing levels are based on objective findings. Although one study (Whitman, Kim, Davidson, Wolf, & Wang, 2002) was unable to link the impact of staffing on two nurse-sensitive clinical outcomes—central line infections and pressure ulcer rates across intensive care and intermediate care units—an inverse link between staffing and patient was found in cardiac intensive care units, medication errors in intensive care units, and restraint rates in medical surgical units. However, actual patient acuity was not considered, which may be a limitation of the study. Another study (Vahey et al., 2004) showed that inadequate staffing accounted for patient dissatisfaction and nurses' emotional exhaustion, which is a component of nurse burnout and is related to nurses leaving the organization.

Compensation

Pay itself is not the major factor in recruiting and retaining the best and the brightest nurses, but monetary reward is an essential component of adequate compensation (Upenieks, 2003). However, tuition reimbursement, on-site academic nursing degree programs, pay for continuing education, and preceptor and charge nurse pay are important to nurses and were included in personnel policies at the hospitals of interviewed CNOs. Nurses rewarded for their contributions to care given during high acuity and nursing shortages, and who are compensated for working extra shifts, do retain their positions in their organizations.

Sick Child and Daycare Services

Organizations that provide on-campus sick child care and extended-hour daycare services offer a tremendous benefit to young nurses who are balancing personal and professional responsibilities (Upenieks, 2003). Nurse retention and engagement are enhanced. Forty percent of nurses chose to leave their positions in one health care system because they needed to provide child or elder care (Strachota et al., 2003).

Role Clarity

Wicker (2004) addressed the need to have clear and specific job descriptions and competencies. Nurses need to know what is expected of them, so that they can perform optimally. Her philosophy is supported by Buckingham and Coffman (1999), who stated that clarifying job expectations is the first job of every manager, if managers expect staff to be fully engaged in the organization.

Several CNOs implemented processes to support staff in successfully achieving national certification by providing in-house preparation courses, paying for certification examinations and, in the case of Aurora Metro, even hosting the exam on-site to minimize test anxiety related to being in a strange place for the test (Golanowski, 2004).

Involvement in Decision-Making

Staff nurse involvement in selecting retention programs was consistently mentioned by the CNOs. Celebrations during Nurses' Week were designed by staff to recognize excellence and were implemented at many of the magnet hospitals. Academic scholarships are awarded during the celebration as well as grants for projects and research activities.

Professional Models of Care: Sensitivity to Values and Preferences of the Organization

Many theories and models are incorporated throughout Magnet facilities. Some are based on published theories and others are based on concepts such as nursing, person, health, and environment described by High Point Regional Health System (ANCC, 2004b). All of the elements in the eight essentials had significant intersections with professional models of care. The Magnet program does not dictate which professional model of care to use. It enables each facility to provide care that meets the needs of the population it serves. The nursing process provides a framework for these models of care. The steps of assessment, diagnosis, outcome identification, planning, implementation, and evaluation serve as the foundation of clinical decision-making and are used to provide evidence-based practice (ANA, 2004).

One early study found that both staff nurses and directors agreed that environment and the practice mode are the two major components making professional nursing practice possible (McClure et al., 1983). This was reinforced by the 2002 study by Kramer and Schmalenberg, which listed control over nursing practice and practice environment as one of the top essentials of a Magnet environment by staff nurses. Magnet hospitals demonstrate control over environment by having nurses in charge of decisions affecting nursing care. Hackensack University Medical Center changed its model to an outcome-based practice, which was also supported by evidence-based management implemented by the Department of Patient Care Council Structure when they restructured the existing nursing councils. Doing this allowed nurses at all levels of patient care to have the responsibility and authority for the delivery of patient care (ANCC, 2004b).

Other key aspects of ensuring professional models of care is to ensure that advanced practice nurses are available to provide patient care as well as consultation to staff nurses. James A. Haley Veteran's Hospital has established a "Nursing Intervention Clinic" that allows nurses to apply the nursing process to assess patients and perform numerous interventions (ANCC, 2004b).

In addition to the care delivery model, this FOM incorporates regulatory considerations and staffing systems. The state Nurse Practice Act and any other state regulatory stipulations should be communicated, understood by all levels of staff, and enforced by nursing leadership at all levels. The CNOs who were interviewed understood the importance of communication at all levels; they provided communication beginning in nursing orientation and continuing throughout employment by rounding, newsletters, electronic bulletin boards, and meetings. They were clear about reinforcing the communications at every level throughout the leadership structure.

Evidence-based staffing systems are also an important component of this force; this is demonstrated by Magnet hospitals in a variety of ways. Key aspects of staffing systems in magnet hospitals tend to be accountability and empowerment by nurses. The University of Kentucky Hospital describes its five-step process that stipulates that the RN knows the expected patient outcomes, determines the resources needed and uses interventions to achieve these outcomes, evaluates progress, and communicates to the next shift (ANCC, 2004b). Nurse-to-patient ratios are not static, but are evaluated using a variety of mechanisms. Kramer and Schmalenberg found that working with other nurses who are clinically competent was the most significantly factor correlating with a perception of adequate staffing, job satisfaction, and perceived ability to give quality care. Furthermore, a close relationship was found between competence and attraction and retention.

Quality Improvement

Quality improvement activities are viewed as educational and nonpunitive. It is generally an integral component of shared governance. Quality improvement efforts in Magnet organizations always include staff nurses and often have them in leadership positions on nursing and multidisciplinary teams. Rebecca Burke at The Miriam Hospital stated, "The key to Magnet is that it is all about the staff nurses at the bedside. Staff nurses make a difference in patient outcomes." At St Joseph's Hospital, quality improvement and evidence-based practice are all linked at the Center for Nursing Excellence. Susan Grant, CNO at the first ANCC-designated Magnet facility, the University of Washington Medical Center (UWMC), said that, "quality is a big one and must be kept at the forefront" (2004). The UWMC Professional and Local Practice Councils integrate evidence-based practice into all dimensions of nursing. Nurses are then encouraged to identify clinical issues and use an evidence-based approach to improve care. Baylor has organized discussions of quality at the unit-level, service line, and in its hospitalwide practice councils (ANCC, 2004b). The ANCC monitors the data collected by Magnet facilities on an annual basis and notifies them about significant events that may cause organizational difficulty in meeting Magnet standards (ANCC, 2004a).

Consultation and Resources

The environment must have adequate internal and external resources to support professional nursing practice as well as show positive results. Extensive use of advanced practice nurses, particularly clinical nurse specialists (CNSs), is described by leaders in many Magnet hospitals. UWMC has centralized Staff Development Specialists and unit-based educators. CNSs provide clinical consultation, direct service, educational offerings, and project development. Fox Chase Cancer Center expands its list of experts available to specially trained pain resources nurses, masters-prepared clinical managers and directors, and peer support from nurses and other disciplines. Middlesex Hospital added a wound and skin team, IV therapy team, infection control liaisons, behavioral health care managers, hospice/palliative care coordinators, and home care cardiac care case management (ANCC, 2004b). Magnet hospitals don't hesitate to get outside help if needed to improve processes. Southwestern Vermont's leadership team partnered to build a culture of empowerment. They reached outside of their organization and hired Porter-O'Grady to assist them to successfully institute shared governance that actively involves physicians. They also collaborated with a local PhD researcher and recruited her as the chair of the research committee (Wicker, 2004). Aurora Health Care, after getting "bogged down" with shared governance, also brought in an expert to help enhance the model and provide input into implementation (Golanowski, 2004). CNO executives recognize the power of bringing in the experts and sometimes get coaching themselves to increase performance. Deb Mals (2004) of Miami Valley Hospital pursued coaching to better manage her calendar. The grueling 14- to 16-hour days that often accompany the CNO job can take their toll, and she realized the importance of being a good role model. Nursing management is not so popular, she reports, but her goal is to have a waiting list for the position of nurse manager; she is taking steps to ensure that nursing directors have the skills to successfully coach and mentor staff nurses (Mals).

Community and the Health Care Organization

UWMC has created a Patient and Family Advisory Council to provide insight and to give input and feedback into programs and delivery of services (ANCC, 2004b). In addition, UWMC partners with community members to provide services to vulnerable populations such as infant mortality prevention services, early post-birth home visitation services, and senior citizen health risk screenings.

Aurora Health Care provides nurse practitioner-led health care clinic services in a grocery store for vulnerable populations (ANCC, 2004b). Hackensack University Medical Center's advance practice nurses make house calls to frail elderly in their community along with other members of the health care team. The program enables patients to remain in their homes for as long as possible before being admitted to the hospital.

Nurses at High Point Regional Health System in North Carolina participate in health fairs that are held twice each year at the local shopping mall. In addition to health education, staff nurses perform blood pressure and blood glucose screenings (ANCC, 2004b). At Holy Cross Hospital in Fort Lauderdale, Florida, staff nurses are involved in parish nursing, school nursing, and HIV/AIDs education. Their Center for Diabetes supports the community through outreach activities (ANCC, 2004b).

RNs at Acadia Hospital in Bangor, Maine, lead community support groups, teach health care workers in group homes and nursing homes, and sit on Mental Health provider boards. Staff nurses volunteer their time along with physicians and other members of the health care team to provide free care for the uninsured in Sioux Falls (ANCC, 2004b).

A final example of a creative way to meet the needs of the health care community was described by Wicker (2004). At a meeting of the Vermont Organizations of Hospitals, the CNO and CEO presented Southwestern Vermont Medical Center's (SVMC's) magnet journey. After the presentation, the CEO offered help free of charge to any other hospital in the state to achieve Magnet designation. Since then, half- and full-day programs have been offered. Hospitals outside of Vermont are charged for the service, and the small consulting practice helps SVMC to continue to grow in expertise. In addition, hospital staff who visit share their creative ideas, which benefits SVMC.

There are many ways for nurses within organizations to support their community's hospitals. They are respected members of the community who are often sought out to raise the level of health awareness of people who are not employed in health care, to give input into community-based projects and programs, and to provide leadership in activities that do relate to health care. Being recognized as a community partner affords hospitals and their staffs the opportunity to influence decisions that do impact the hospital and its operation. The above descriptions of several hospitals' projects are included as only a few examples of community involvement.

Nurses as Teachers

Many magnet facilities identified the following list of education-related activities as most common in the organization (ANCC, 2004b). Nurses serve as preceptors to new staff, trainers for life support classes, instructors for continuing education, clinical instructors for students, and facilitators for patient education. Advance practice nurses teach academic courses and oversee groups of students in the clinical setting.

Teaching is a hallmark of nursing practice. The nurse's role as teacher begins with the patient in the bed or in the clinic and moves to the novice new graduate and student nurses, to the manager interested in learning more about a new protocol or care of a complex patient, to members of the interdisciplinary team, to hospital leaders who need to learn about the practice environment or culture, all the way to members of the Board of Directors who will be making decisions that ultimately impact nurses' day-to-day work. In addition, teaching extends to community organizations such as schools and churches. Nurses teach by way of publishing new knowledge gained from research activities and by sharing their wisdom in academic classes, conferences, or workshops. These examples of teaching illustrate the vast impact that nurses have on their environment as well as different populations.

Northeast Medical Center in Concord, North Carolina, provides a unique teaching opportunity to staff nurses at the annual nursing camp offered to high school students interested in nursing as a career (ANCC, 2004b). Middlesex Hospital in Connecticut offers a one-year Residency Program for new RN graduates that is taught by expert staff nurses.

Moore described a unique teaching opportunity that has evolved over the past few years. Nurses from hospitals in four Caribbean countries come to Atlanta to learn to how to implement Magnet concepts within their own hospitals and countries. St. Joseph's nurses are preparing to visit their sister facilities to teach oncology content, and the foreign nurses will come to St. Joseph's to observe and be precepted in chemotherapy administration.

Image of Nursing

The image of nursing reflects the degree to which nurses' professional colleagues, including physicians, view the role of nursing as integral to the overall operation and survival of the hospital (ANCC, 2004a). Nursing's active participation in organizational decision-making is essential if nursing is to influence the delivery of patient care. At SVMC, the CEO reinforced the importance of nursing when he stated that the role of the hospital was to take care of patients, and since nurses drive the culture of patient care and coordinate the care, he would support implementation of the newly proposed nursing shared governance model (Wicker, 2004). His message was clear and his belief in the necessity of nursing as the driver of the care left no room for misunderstanding or confusion.

An example from the literature provides an innovative example of a regulatory approach to demonstrate professional competence, credibility, and value. Professional certification of nurses in Russia requires recertification every five years; at this time, the level of professional qualification is assigned by specialty as well as a commensurate pay scale (Weinstein & Antonova, 2003). There are 16 specialties and 18 pay categories. This system of certification by specialty and recertification that is ongoing may be evidence of the value placed on the unique body of knowledge by clinical specialty required to care for various populations of patients. By recognizing individual specialties and levels of qualification, staffing guidelines must be addressed as well as floating expectations. These directly influence the image of nursing.

Golanowski (2004) provided several examples of nursing's influence at the organizational level. First, staff nurses attend Medical Executive Committee meetings. Second, the chair of the System Shared Governance Council is a voting member of the system CNO group. Third, meetings to address clinical safety issues are scheduled around caregivers' schedules, including nurses' schedules, so that they can participate even if they are on the night shift (ANCC, 2004b).

At Avera McKennan Hospital & University Health Center, 16 nurses were recognized at the regional or national level for excellence in nursing in 2004, which strongly contributes to the image of nursing (ANCC, 2004b). The Tampa Bay community voted Bayfront Medical Center the "Best Nursing Staff in the Tampa Bay Area," with an accompanying article published in the *Medical Newspaper*, and the *Advance for Nurses Magazine* awarded the hospital's ICU nursing staff as the Best Nursing Team in the State of Florida (ANCC, 2004b). Cedars-Sinai has established the Institute for Professional Nursing Development, which offers a wide array of programs for nurses (ANCC, 2004b).

At St. Joseph's Hospital, staff were concerned with their professional image and patients' perceptions of them. They surveyed staff nurses, asking questions about personal appearance and interactions with patients. Results of the survey indicated that staff introduced themselves to patients, gave their phone numbers, and wrote their names on the patients' dry erase boards. Nurses also indicated that they enjoyed wearing different colors and did not believe that the colors were unprofessional. Nurses next conducted a survey to learn patients' perceptions of nurses' attire. Seven hundred patients were surveyed. Patients stated that they liked seeing nurses in different colors because it made things more interesting, but if nurses had to wear one color, the patients preferred blue. The Shared Governance Council compiled the information and made a recommendation to the executive team, which was to allow nurses to wear colors of their choice along with either a blue or white lab coat or jacket containing the hospital logo and RN credentials. The executive team accepted the recommendation and paid for lab coat monogramming for staff who bought jackets. All chose blue or white jackets (Moore, 2004).

Linda Deering (2004), CNO at Delnor Community Hospital, summed up the concept of image of nursing when she said that, "self esteem is critical. One's personal demeanor, if not positive, prevents others from respecting you. It is necessary for nurses to understand their role in the organization and the impact they make on patient care."

Interdisciplinary Relationships

According to Wicker (2004), "nursing staff identify that the number one factor that keeps them at SVMC is that they are respected members of the health care team and that they are colleagues with physicians." They are equal members on the team. They are integral in developing the patient's plan of care and jointly develop goals to support the patient.

Golanowski (2004) described a strategy that was implemented to recognize positive RN–physician relationships. The nursing department initiated an annual "Physician of the Year" award to recognize collaborative practice. The CNO presented the new award program to Medical Executive Committee. At first, it was met with lukewarm enthusiasm. RNs nominate physicians by writing a narrative of a situation in which the physician worked collaboratively with a nurse to affect a positive patient outcome. A panel of nurses reviews the narratives and selects one physician. Over the course of the five years that physicians have been recognized, there is growing interest on the part of the physicians, and several have asked for the criteria for selection. They understand that it is not a popularity contest and are interested in being recognized for their collaborative practice. Staff nurses now sit on several medical staff committees, including Medical Executive, Quality Council, and the Safety Committee. These nurses speak up and address committee members as colleagues. The CNO has joined the NPC and attends monthly meetings on an ongoing basis.

Deering (2004) provided great insight into the relationships between nurses and physicians in the following paragraph.

The goal is to be collegial. Collegial relationships require overt discussion about patients' plans of care. Nurses need to use professional language. As nurses become nationally certified and obtain their BSNs, they will gain more confidence and behaviors will change and become more collegial. It is important for nurses to manage up. For example, rather than telling a patient, "I have no idea when your physician will be here," say, "Let me call your physician's office to see when he is scheduled to be here today." At Delnor we did not focus on physician behavior; instead, we focused on our own behavior. We asked what makes us valuable and respected. We stopped discrediting ourselves. For example, when asked by a physician, how is my patient doing? Responding with "I don't know. I just got here," discredits the nurse. Telling the physician, "Here's what I do know from report and I'd like to go on rounds with you and talk to the patient," is collaborative and supports movement to collegial. If nurses would view physicians as our primary customer by responding to their needs and giving them quality information in a timely manner, we would strengthen our relationships.

The nurse–physician relationship is the most important relationship in an environment that supports professional nursing practice, as reported in the literature as well as with the CNOs who were interviewed for this chapter. Kramer and Schmalenberg (2002) used mutual respect, interdependency, concern for patients, and good communication as the descriptors of collaborative practice. Working together to set goals and plan patients' care results in a positive work environment, one in which nurses feel respected and recognized for their expertise (Upenieks, 2003). Vahey and colleagues (2004) reported that poor nurse–physician relationships accounted for patient dissatisfaction and nurses' emotional exhaustion, which is a component of nurse burnout, leading to their desire to leave the organization.

Professional Development

Professional development has several components, including orientation, continuing education, formal education, and career development (ANCC, 2004b). Adequate financial support of these important components is evident in the Magnet organizations' budgets. Availability of easily accessible academic programs is found as well as many on-site BSN and MSN programs to support career advancement opportunities. Educators, CNSs, and other education resources are also available to support staff along their professional development journeys.

Leadership competencies are essential to empower nurses in a variety of situations from the bedside to the conference room. Malloch (2003) reported on the Arizona Nurse Leadership model, which was developed to support the practice of bedside caregivers. Two of these competencies—interpersonal and technical—

were identified by several of the interviewed CNOs. Team building and conflict management are two skills of interpersonally competent nurses. These skills facilitate nurses' communication with members of the interdisciplinary team as well as prepare them to be effective members of shared governance councils, and other unit and hospital-based committees and teams.

Upenieks (2003) identified available continuing education and tailored comprehensive orientation programs as two vital components of a professional practice environment. Several of the CNOs endorsed continuing education and orientation. They also included the necessity of formal orientation to new members of shared governance councils. Gokenbach at William Beaumont Hospital shared her strategy to establish an evidence-based culture through in-depth training of unit level staff to become unit-based researchers. A doctorally prepared nurse researcher meets formally with these staff members to teach them the skills of conducting literature searches, selecting best practices, and then evaluating and using them. Staff nurses are then invited to attend the hospital's annual Research Conference.

Working with nurses who are clinically competent is one of the essentials of magnetism identified by Kramer and Schmalenberg (2002). To ensure that nurses are clinically competent, Magnet facilities have implemented a variety of programs. For example, at University of Washington Medical Center, a New Graduate Residency Program and a Perioperative Internship are offered to prepare new nurses to meet clinical performance expectations in their respective clinical specialty (ANCC, 2004b).

Aurora Health Care Metro Region has developed a professional development model using a peer review process based on Patricia Benner's novice-to-expert continuum (ANCC, 2004b). This model measures and recognizes nurses' experience, knowledge, and skills related to patient care. Nursing education specialist positions were created to support the organization's commitment to life-long learning.

SUMMARY

Evidence-based practice uses the best research with clinical expertise and patient values. As Magnet hospitals mature in their roles and the FOM continue to grow, we continually see creativity in delivering quality care and a passionate drive toward excellence. The strong relationship between the FOM and the Eight Essentials of Magnetism as perceived by staff nurses in the literature and the CNOs interviewed in this chapter provides the basis for the excellence in nursing that is well documented in Magnet hospitals. This does not mean that once a facility is designated a Magnet, it will always maintain those credentials.

Magnet designation requires persistent development of evidence-based practices, evolving programs of excellence, and an ability to bring the ideal future to the present reality. Some facilities may not be able to continue the rigorous pace and will lose their designation, or simply choose to not redesignate for a variety of reasons. An episode may occur that is so severe that an organization may have the designation revoked. Losing the designation not by choice has occurred twice in the history of the program (*American Journal of Nursing,* 2003).

The increased growth of the program reached a tipping point in 2003 and continues to gain prestige as it expands in number. *U.S. News and World Report* recently included Magnet designation in the criteria for its annual "100 Best Hospital" list, and 43% of the facilities named on the list were Magnet-designated facilities (*U.S. News and World* Report, 2004). This is significant, since the current roster of Magnets comprise only 2% of the nation's approximate 5,794 hospitals (AHA Hospital Statistics, 2004). Hospitals choosing to take the Magnet journey invest a significant amount of resources into the development of the culture, but once they reach the pinnacle of success, they always say it was worth the journey.

REFERENCES

Aiken, L., Clarke, S., Cheung, R., Sloane, D., & Silber, J. (2003). Educational levels of hospital nurses and surgical patient mortality. *Journal of the American Medical Association, 290*(12), 1617–1623.

American Journal of Nursing. (2003). Editorial: Winning and losing Magnet designation, the ANCC gets tough. *103*(5), 25.

American Hospital Statistics: AMA website, ANA resource center; Fast Facts from AHA Hospital statistics; Available at http://www.aha.org/aha/resource_center/fastfacts/fast_facts_US_hosptals.html.

American Nurses Association. (2004). *Nursing: Scope and Standards of Practice.* Washington, DC: American Nurses Publishing.

American Nurses Association. (1991). *Standards for Organized Nursing Services and Responsibilities of Nurse Administrators Across All Settings.* Washington, DC: American Nurses Publishing.

American Nurses Credentialing Center. (2003). *Magnet Recognition Program Recognizing Excellence in Nursing Service: Health Care Instructions and Application Process Manual,* 2002–2004 edition. Available at http://www.nursecredentialing.org. Accessed March 2005.

American Nurses Credentialing Center. (2004a). Magnet Recognition Program Application Manual, 2005 edition. Silver Spring, MD: ANCC.

American Nurses Credentialing Center. (2004b). Magnet: Best Practices in Today's Challenging Health Care Environment. Silver Spring, MD: ANCC.

Buckingham, M., & Coffman, C. (1999). *First, Break All the Rules: What the World's Greatest Managers Do Differently.* New York, NY: Simon & Schuster.

Burke, R. (2004). Magnet CNO Interview. Personal communication, The Miriam Hospital, Providence, RI.

Collins, J. (2001). *Good to Great: Why Some Companies Make the Leap and Others Don't.* New York, NY: HarperCollins Publishers, Inc.

Deering, L. (2004). Magnet CNO Interview. Personal communication, Delnor Community Hospital, Geneva, IL.

Fiore, T. (2004). Magnet CNO Interview. Personal communication, Hackensack Hospital, Hackensack, NJ.

Gokenbach, V. (2004). Magnet CNO Interview. Personal communication, William Beaumont Hospital, Royal Oak, MI.

Golanowski, M. (2004). Magnet CNO Interview. Personal communication, Aurora Health Care, Metro Region, WI.

Grant, S. (2004). Magnet CNO Interview. Personal communication. The University of Washington Medical Center, Seattle, WA.

Hader, R. (2004). Nursing Management Congress 2004. Presentation: The Forces of Magnetism. Chicago, IL.

Havens, D. S., & Vasey, J. (2003). Measuring staff nurse decisional involvement: The decisional involvement scale. *Journal of Nursing Administration, 33*(6), 331–336.

Horton-Deutsch, S. L., & Wellman, D. S. (2002). Christman's principles for effective management: Reflection and challenges for action. *Journal of Nursing Administration, 32*(11), 596–601.

Kleinman, C. S. (2004). Leadership and retention: Research needed. *Journal of Nursing Administration, 34*(3), 111–113.

Kramer, M., & Schmalenberg, C. (2002). Staff nurses identify essentials of magnetism. In M. McClure & A. S. Hinshaw (Ed.), *Magnet Hospitals Revisited: Attraction and Retention of Professional Nurses.* Washington, DC: American Nurses Publishing, 25–59, 31–34.

Luzinski, C. (2004). Magnet CNO Interview. Personal communication, Poudre Valley Health System, Ft. Collins, CO.

Malloch, K. (2003, April 1). Leadership model: Leadership model focuses on RN's authoritative role to boost uniformity, job satisfaction. Available at http://www.NurseWeek.com/news/features/03-04/models_print.html. Accessed March 2005.

Mals, D. (2004). Magnet CNO Interview. Personal communication, Miami Valley Hospital, Dayton, OH.

Marx, D. (2001, April 17). Medical event reporting system – transfusion medicine (MERS-TM). In *Patient Safety and the "Just Culture:" A Primer for Health Care Executives.* Funded by a grant from the National Heart, Lung and Blood Institute, National Institutes of Health; 1–28. Available at http://www.mers-tm.net/support/Marx_Primer.pdf. Accessed March 2005.

McClure, M. L., & Hinshaw, A. S. (2002). *Magnet Hospitals Revisited: Attraction and Retention of Professional Nurses.* Washington, DC: American Nurses Publishing.

McClure, M.M., Poulin, M., Sovie, M., & Wandelt, M. (1983). *Magnet Hospitals: Attraction and Retention of Professional Nurses.* American Academy of Nursing Task Force on Nursing Practice in Hospitals. Kansas City, MO: American Nurses Association.

Moore, V. (2004). Magnet CNO Interview. Personal Communication, St. Joseph's, Atlanta, GA.

Neuhauser, P. C. (2002). Building a high-retention culture in healthcare: Fifteen ways to get good people to stay. *Journal of Nursing Administration, 32*(9), 470–478.

Pekkanen, J. (2003, September). Condition: Critical. *Reader's Digest,* 84–93.

Porter-O'Grady, T. (2003). Researching shared governance: A futility of focus. *Journal of Nursing Administration, 33*(4), 251–252.

Strachota, E., Normandin, P., O'Brien, N., Clary, M., & Krukow, B. (2003). Reasons registered nurses leave or change employment status. *Journal of Nursing Administration, 33*(2), 111–117.

Tonges, M. C., Baloga-Altieri, B., & Atzori, M. (2004). Amplifying nursing's voice through a staff-management partnership. *Journal of Nursing Administration, 34*(3), 134–139.

University of South Florida. (2004). Research and Practice Program Guide. In 1st Annual Florida Magnet Nursing Research Conference. Available at http://www.research.usf.edu/absolutenm/templates/newro.asp?articleid=166&zoneid=2. Accessed March 2005.

Upenieks, V. V. (2003). What constitutes effective leadership? Perceptions of magnet and nonmagnet nurse leaders. *Journal of Nursing Administration, 32*(9), 456–467.

U.S. News and World Report. (2004, July 12). America's Best Hospitals: The Honor Roll. Available at http:www.usnews.com. Accessed March 2005.

Vahey, D. C., Aiken, L. H., Sloane, D., Clarke, S. P., & Vargas, D. (2004). Nurse burnout and patient satisfaction. *Medical Care, 42*(2, suppl II), II-57–II-66.

Weinstein, S. M., & Antonova, S. (2003). Enhancing nurse-physician collaboration: A staffing innovation. *Journal of Nursing Administration, 33*(4), 193–195.

Wicker, M. (2004). Magnet CNO Interview. Personal communication, Southwestern Vermont Medical Center, Bennington, VT.

Whitman, G. R., Kim, Y., Davidson, L. J., Wolf, G. A., & Wang, S. L. (2002). The impact of staffing on patient outcomes across specialty units. *Journal of Nursing Administration, 32*(12), 633–639.

Index